P9-CRC-438

Preserving Public Trust:

Accreditation and Human Research Participant Protection Programs

Committee on Assessing the System for Protecting Human
Research Subjects

Board on Health Sciences Policy

INSTITUTE OF MEDICINE

NATIONAL ACADEMY PRESS
Washington, D.C.

NATIONAL ACADEMY PRESS • **2101 Constitution Avenue, N.W.** • **Washington, DC 20418**

NOTICE: The project that is the subject of this report was approved by the Governing Board of the National Research Council, whose members are drawn from the councils of the National Academy of Sciences, the National Academy of Engineering, and the Institute of Medicine. The members of the committee responsible for the report were chosen for their special competences and with regard for appropriate balance.

This project, N01-OD-4-2139, Task Order No. 80, received support from the evaluation set-aside Section 513, Public Health Service Act. The U.S. Department of Health and Human Services provided this support, with additional support provided by the Greenwall Foundation. The views presented in this report are those of the Institute of Medicine Committee on Assessing the System for Protecting Human Research Subjects and are not necessarily those of the funding agencies.

International Book Standard No. 0-309-07328-6

Additional copies of this report are available for sale from the National Academy Press, 2101 Constitution Avenue, N.W., Box 285, Washington, D.C. 20055. Call (800) 624-6242 or (202) 334-3313 (in the Washington metropolitan area), or visit the NAP's home page at **www.nap.edu.** The full text of this report is available at **www.nap.edu.**

For more information about the Institute of Medicine, visit the IOM home page at **www.iom.edu.**

"Knowing is not enough; we must apply.
Willing is not enough; we must do."

—Goethe

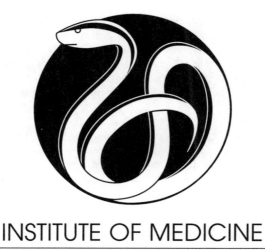

INSTITUTE OF MEDICINE

Shaping the Future for Health

THE NATIONAL ACADEMIES

National Academy of Sciences
National Academy of Engineering
Institute of Medicine
National Research Council

The **National Academy of Sciences** is a private, nonprofit, self-perpetuating society of distinguished scholars engaged in scientific and engineering research, dedicated to the furtherance of science and technology and to their use for the general welfare. Upon the authority of the charter granted to it by the Congress in 1863, the Academy has a mandate that requires it to advise the federal government on scientific and technical matters. Dr. Bruce M. Alberts is president of the National Academy of Sciences.

The **National Academy of Engineering** was established in 1964, under the charter of the National Academy of Sciences, as a parallel organization of outstanding engineers. It is autonomous in its administration and in the selection of its members, sharing with the National Academy of Sciences the responsibility for advising the federal government. The National Academy of Engineering also sponsors engineering programs aimed at meeting national needs, encourages education and research, and recognizes the superior achievements of engineers. Dr. William A. Wulf is president of the National Academy of Engineering.

The **Institute of Medicine** was established in 1970 by the National Academy of Sciences to secure the services of eminent members of appropriate professions in the examination of policy matters pertaining to the health of the public. The Institute acts under the responsibility given to the National Academy of Sciences by its congressional charter to be an adviser to the federal government and, upon its own initiative, to identify issues of medical care, research, and education. Dr. Kenneth I. Shine is president of the Institute of Medicine.

The **National Research Council** was organized by the National Academy of Sciences in 1916 to associate the broad community of science and technology with the Academy's purposes of furthering knowledge and advising the federal government. Functioning in accordance with general policies determined by the Academy, the Council has become the principal operating agency of both the National Academy of Sciences and the National Academy of Engineering in providing services to the government, the public, and the scientific and engineering communities. The Council is administered jointly by both Academies and the Institute of Medicine. Dr. Bruce M. Alberts and Dr. William A. Wulf are chairman and vice chairman, respectively, of the National Research Council.

COMMITTEE ON ASSESSING THE SYSTEM FOR PROTECTING HUMAN RESEARCH SUBJECTS

DANIEL D. FEDERMAN (*Chair*), Senior Dean for Alumni Relations and Clinical Teaching, Harvard University, Boston, MA

DANIEL AZARNOFF, President, D.L. Azarnoff Associates, San Francisco, CA, and Vice President of Clinical and Regulatory Affairs, Cellegy Pharmaceuticals

TOM BEAUCHAMP, Professor, Kennedy Institute of Ethics, Georgetown University, Washington, DC

TIMOTHY STOLTZFUS JOST, Newton D. Baker-Baker and Hostetler Professor of Law and Health Services Management and Policy, Ohio State University, Columbus, OH

PATRICIA A. KING, Carmack Waterhouse Professor of Law, Medicine, Ethics, and Public Policy, Georgetown University Law Center, Washington, DC

RODERICK J.A. LITTLE, Chair, Department of Biostatistics, School of Public Health, University of Michigan, Ann Arbor, MI

JAMES McNULTY, President, Depressive/Manic Depressive Association of Rhode Island, Bristol, RI

ANNE PETERSEN, Senior Vice President-Programs, Kellogg Foundation, Battle Creek, MI

BONNIE W. RAMSEY, Professor, Department of Pediatrics, University of Washington School of Medicine, Seattle, WA

LYDIA VILLA-KOMAROFF, Vice President for Research, Northwestern University, Evanston, IL

FRAN VISCO, President, The National Breast Cancer Coalition, Washington, DC

Expert Advisers

KAY DICKERSIN, Associate Professor, Department of Community Health, Brown University, Providence, RI

ALBERTO GRIGNOLO, Senior Vice President and General Manager for Worldwide Regulatory Affairs, PAREXEL International, Waltham, MA

MARY FAITH MARSHALL, Professor of Medicine, School of Medicine, Kansas University Medical Center, Kansas City, KS

CAROL SAUNDERS, President, Center for Clinical Research Practice, Wellesley, MA

DENNIS TOLSMA, Director, Clinical Quality Improvement, Kaiser Permanente, Atlanta, GA

Liaisons

RICHARD J. BONNIE, John S. Battle Professor of Law and Director, Institute of Law, Psychiatry, and Public Policy, Charlottesville, VA

Preface

Although it is said that each stage of evolution can be explained (but not predicted) from the earlier ones, it is not easy to apply this insight to the specifically human phenomenon known as clinical investigation. With the possible exception of genes for altruism, it is hard to discern the evolutionary antecedents of the behaviors that characterize what we know as human research. The complex system that sustains research is ultimately premised on trust—trust in the people and organizations that conduct research. In the wake of revelations about lapses in research ethics, such trust must be earned, and trust hinges on concrete affirmation of trustworthiness. But trustworthiness to whom? To those who become the object of study in human research.

Consider first those who join the human research system as participants. Those who are volunteers have little to gain by accepting drugs or answering a survey, each of which has a small but unquantified risk. Although a financial inducement is sometimes part of the lure, these individuals often accept considerable risk in the knowledge that the research in which they join cannot help them but does have the potential to help "unknown others"—surely a remarkably selfless behavior. The other key participants are patients who become the subject of research. At some point, all new drugs and devices are given experimentally to sick individuals who might benefit from the intervention. Even when they are explicitly informed of the relative risks and benefits, many patients choose to enroll in a clinical investigation when their own likelihood of benefiting is small. The outcome of this moment of decision affects in considerable measure how the clinician/researcher discharges his or her responsibility to inform.

Protecting research participants looms especially large in clinical research, where the risks are often the highest, professional roles are conflicted, and ethical lapses have been most salient. The physician doing research is wittingly cast in two different and often conflicting roles. Above all else, he or she is a doctor, sworn first to do no harm and always to act in the best interest of the patient. As investigator, however, the same person is trained to randomize his or her patient's participation to an at least 50 percent likelihood of no benefit and, indeed, to treat all research participants with a neutral regard that puts the sought-after truth ahead of the research participant's immediate interest. As if this dual identity of dedicated physician and disinterested inquirer were not enough of a weight to sustain, the physician researcher has two burdens of (self) interest. One of these, familiar now for more than half a century, is the linkage of research and publication to academic promotion and professional advancement. The other, newer pressure is that of obtaining additional income from sources that have a huge interest in a positive outcome of the research. Many and perhaps most clinical trials are now supported by pharmaceutical and biotechnology companies. Honoraria, speaker fees, paid travel, and further research support may all be available to the bearer of positive tidings. These emoluments, though, are dwarfed by the potential of equity participation in the sponsoring company by the investigator.

The social and economic setting of research also is undergoing dramatic change. At first investigation was almost an avocation of scientists and clinicians whose curiosity and clinically derived puzzlement drove them to undertake a study. Later it was a virtual monopoly of academic health centers, where a dominant professional ethos and the constant gaze of skeptical trainees emphasized probity and ethics. In the 1970s, institutional review boards (IRBs) became increasingly common, applying independent review and intellectual rigor to the evaluation of the science and the protection of the individual subject participants. Now, however, clinical research is a multibillion dollar business with enormous potential profits riding on efficiency, aggressiveness, and positive outcomes. Research pervades marketing, census counting, national surveys of opinion, and myriad other aspects of our daily lives. Outputs of research define congressional districts, legal thresholds for poverty, and marketing campaigns that affect us all. Research is carried out in a ragged congeries of universities, for-profit and nonprofit research organizations, and drug companies. Reassurance about the conduct of some of research comes from professional independent review boards that have no anchor in universities or their academic health centers and that are often organized for profit.

As a result of these changes plus the headlong advance in biomedical science, questions are surfacing around the enterprise and about its dedication to the human being at its center—the research participant. Given the complexity of the current science, can consent ever be truly informed? Given the inevitable asymmetry of the investigator-subject dyad, can real autonomy—the power to say no and the choice to change one's mind—be preserved? Can IRBs of such different geneses handle the complex responsibilities being laid on them? Can professionalism be sustained without requiring saintliness? Can the occasional sinner be recognized before doing tragic harm? In short, how can a diffuse, chaotic, fast-moving, ever-changing nonsystem of evolutionarily unprecedented human behavior be organized and monitored to maximize its glorious potential and control its dark risks?

Our committee was asked to take up these questions and others with the focus on the safety and rights of the participants who share the clinical research enterprise and who are indispensable to its success. In this first report, done in 6 months, we suggest ways in which accreditation might contribute to a new level of excellence. There are many other points of leverage, however, including decompressing the burdens on IRBs, educating and perhaps certifying investigators, improving research monitoring, and building greater institutional support and infrastructure. In another report to be rendered after more time, more study, and more reflection, we hope to contribute to these larger questions and thus to the research enterprise as a social good.

Daniel D. Federman, M.D., Chair

REVIEWERS

This report has been reviewed in draft form by individuals chosen for their diverse perspectives and technical expertise, in accordance with procedures approved by the NRC's Report Review Committee. The purpose of this independent review is to provide candid and critical comments that will assist the institution in making its published report as sound as possible and to ensure that the report meets institutional standards for objectivity, evidence, and responsiveness to the study charge. The review comments and draft manuscript remain confidential to protect the integrity of the deliberative process. We wish to thank the following individuals for their review of this report:

Eugene Braunwald, Partners HealthCare System
Bette-Jane Crigger, The Hastings Center, *IRB*
Norman Daniels, Tufts University, Department of Community Medicine
Ralph Dell, National Research Council
Janice Douglas-Baltimore, Case Western Reserve University, School of Medicine
Frederick L. Grinnell, University of Texas, Southwestern Medical Center
Eugene Hammel, University of California, Berkeley, Department of Demography
Erica Heath, Independent Review Consulting, Inc.
John G. Miller, Association for Assessment and Accreditation of Laboratory Animal Care
Jonathan D. Moreno, University of Virginia, Center for Biomedical Ethics
Thomas Puglisi, Pricewaterhouse Coopers, LLP
John Sever, Children's National Medical Center
Michael Silverstein, University of Chicago, Department of Anthropology
Eve Slater, Merck & Co., Inc.

Although the reviewers listed above have provided many constructive comments and suggestions, they were not asked to endorse the conclusions or recommendations nor did they see the final draft of the report before its release. The review of this report was overseen by Francois Abboud, appointed by the Institute of Medicine, and Mary Jane Osborn, University of Connecticut Health Center, appointed by the NRC's Report Review Committee, who were responsible for making certain that an independent examination of this report was carried out in accordance with institutional procedures and that all review comments were carefully considered. Responsibility for the final content of this report rests entirely with the authoring committee and the institution.

Acronyms

AAALAC   Association for Assessment and Accreditation of Laboratory
Animal Care

AAHRPP   Association for the Accreditation of Human Research Protection
Programs

AAMC   Association of American Medical Colleges

ACHRE   Advisory Committee on Human Radiation Experiments

AMA   American Medical Association

CIOMS   Council for International Organizations of Medical Sciences

DHHS   U.S. Department of Health and Human Services

DSMBs   data safety and monitoring boards

FDA   Food and Drug Administration

GAO   General Accounting Office

HCFA   Health Care Financing Administration

HRPP   human research protection program

HRPPP   human research participant protection program

ICH-GCP   International Conference on Harmonisation Guideline for Good
Clinical Practice

IND   investigational new drug application (FDA)

IOM   Institute of Medicine

IRB   institutional review board

JCAHO   Joint Commission on Accreditation of Healthcare Organizations

MCMC   Medical Care Management Corporation

MCOs   managed care organizations

NBAC	National Bioethics Advisory Commission
NCI	National Cancer Institute
NCQA	National Committee for Quality Assurance
NHRPAC	National Human Research Protections Advisory Committee
NIH	National Institutes of Health
OHRP	Office for Human Research Protections
OIG	Office of the Inspector General (U.S. Department of Health and Human Services)
OPRR	(former) Office for Protection from Research Risks
ORCA	Office of Research Compliance and Assurance (VA)
PHS	U.S. Public Health Service
PRIM&R	Public Responsibility in Medicine and Research
VA	U.S. Department of Veterans Affairs

Contents

LIST OF TABLES, FIGURES, AND BOXES

Tables

Figures

Boxes

Executive Summary

ABSTRACT

In response to a request from the Secretary of Health and Human Services, the Institute of Medicine formed the Committee on Assessing the System for Protecting Human Research Subjects to conduct a two-phase study to examine how to improve the structure and function of human research review programs. This report provides the committee's response to the tasks in phase 1. With respect to human research review programs, those tasks are to review and consider proposed performance standards, recommend standards for accreditation, and recommend an approach to monitoring and evaluating the system for protection of human research participants. The committee reviewed and considered available draft standards developed independently by Public Responsibility in Medicine and Research (PRIM&R) and the National Committee for Quality Assurance (NCQA), which is under contract to the U.S. Department of Veterans Affairs (VA). The committee provides a series of findings and recommendations for using performance standards to improve the system for protection of human research participants.

The committee finds that the standards proposed by NCQA for VA facilities appear promising for use in the accreditation of VA facilities. The committee regards the standards prepared by NCQA to be more suitable than those prepared by PRIM&R for not only pilot testing in VA facilities but also, with modification, for the accreditation of other research institutions. The NCQA standards are the strongest basis for use in the accreditation of other research institutions because they pay specific attention to quality improvement, provide flexibility in achieving performance goals (e.g., increased protection of research participants), and are explicit in their grounding in current regulations.

The committee recommends that pilot accreditation programs should start from the accreditation standards and processes proposed by NCQA for VA facilities and be adapted for use in other organizational contexts by NCQA or other accreditation bodies. In expanding the draft NCQA accreditation standards for use beyond VA facilities, the committee recommends that the standards be strengthened in several specific ways. These include how investigators will be reviewed, beyond the review of protocols by institutional review boards; how sponsors will be assessed; how participants will be involved in setting performance standards; and how oversight mechanisms can ensure participants' safety.

The committee further recommends that (1) the organizations formulating accreditation standards and carrying out the accreditation process be independent, nongovernmental organizations; (2) the formulation of accreditation standards, the accreditation process, and human research participant protection program operations directly involve research participants; and (3) the accreditation process accommodate organizations involved in research beyond the traditional models of academic health centers and VA facilities and be appropriate for research methods other than clinical research.

Only by experience gained through pilot testing can the value that accreditation adds to the current regulatory system, in terms of enhanced protection of human research participants, be adequately assessed.

Beginning in the 1960s, a formal system for ensuring the ethical conduct of research with humans developed in the United States. This system traditionally centered on the institutional review board (IRB). However, the Committee on Assessing the System for Protecting Human Research Subjects and others now envision a broader system with multiple functional elements that will be referred to in this report as *human research participant protection programs* (HRPPPs) (Figure 1). That system is the central element for protecting the interests of those who participate in research, and it has four principal functions: (1) to ensure that research design is sound and that a study's promise for augmenting knowledge justifies the involvement of human participants,[1] (2) to assess the risks and benefits independently of the investigators who carry out the research; (3) to ensure that participation is voluntary and informed; and (4) to ensure that participants are recruited equitably and that risks and benefits are fairly distributed.

---

[1] See Chapter 1 for discussion regarding the committee's use of the term "participant" versus "subject."

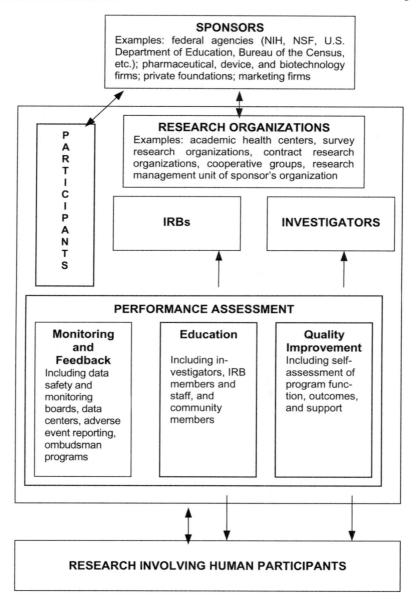

FIGURE 1 Human research participant protection programs. The components in the large box are all parts of an HRPPP. Arrows represent information flow pathways, not organizational responsibilities. All units within an HRPPP should have formalized communication procedures.

When the original system for the protection of human participants in research was created, the typical study was done at a single research institution by a single investigator or a small team of investigators. IRBs[2] were formed to ensure an independent review of proposed research by volunteers at individual sites and remain the centerpiece of HRPPPs. Today, however, some clinical trials involve scores or even hundreds of centers and tens of thousands of participants. With the dramatic increase in privately funded research, a separate system of independent IRBs has also been created; such IRBs typically have professional staff, and their members are often paid for their time and effort. The review system as a whole, however, has not transformed or adapted to the vast growth in the scale and complexity of research.

Research carries with it inherent risk, but it must always be conducted so that risk to research participants is reduced to the minimum necessary and the rights of the volunteers who participate in the research are respected by the entire system of research sponsors, institutions, and investigators (the HRPPP). Trust in the human research enterprise, embodied in an individual consenting to participate in a study, demands that the system responsible for protection be credible and accountable. Yet, the repeated documentation of serious strains on the system has not led to discernible improvement as weaknesses and lapses continue to come to light.

The need to improve HRPPPs has become ever more apparent as report after report highlighting mounting concerns about the ability of HRPPPs to keep up with the evolving research enterprise has been issued (see Chapters 1 and 2). Nearly all of these reports have recommended a reexamination and modernization of the system. In addition, beginning in May 1999, the federal Office for Protection from Research Risks (OPRR) and the Food and Drug Administration (FDA) took action against several major research universities, suspending their human research programs because of apparent noncompliance with federal regulations. In September 1999, Jesse Gelsinger, an 18-year-old research volunteer, died in a gene transfer trial not because of his underlying disease but because of the experimental intervention itself. As the circumstances and events leading up to his death emerged, it became apparent that the system intended to protect him from unacceptable risks in research instead failed him.

In response to these and other events over the last several years, the U.S. Congress, the U.S. Department of Veterans Affairs (VA), and the U.S. Depart-

---

[2] IRBs are defined in federal regulations governing human research (45 CFR 46.107–109; 45 CFR 56.102 (g)). Food and Drug Administration (FDA) regulations cover "independent" IRBs that review privately funded research. The majority of IRBs operate under one or both sets of federal regulations. Some nongovernmental organizations have formed groups to review and approve research that is not subject to federal regulation. These groups can perform the functions of an IRB overseen by FDA or the Office for Human Research Protections (OHRP) but do so outside the purview of FDA and OHRP.

ment of Health and Human Services (DHHS) began looking at how the system for the protection of participants in human research could be brought into line with the new challenges that it faced without unduly limiting opportunities for advancing knowledge through innovative research. In spring 2000, congressional hearings, legislation, and new initiatives announced by the Secretary of Health and Human Services and the VA sought to assure the public that policy makers were aware of the fundamental need to ensure access to the great potential offered by research without sacrificing participant safety or well-being. Likewise, organizations within the research community responded to public concern by reaffirming their commitment to the safe and ethical pursuit of research and by establishing focused task forces to examine identified areas of concern (AAMC et al., 2000; AAU Task Force on Research Accountability, 2000; AAUP, forthcoming) Accreditation of HRPPPs was one of the ideas that emerged from these discussions.

THE COMMITTEE'S TASK

One component of the DHHS effort to examine the system for the protection of human research participants was to ask the Institute of Medicine (IOM) to initiate an in-depth study of how to improve the structure and function of activities related to the protection of participants in human research, with an emphasis on the responsibilities and elements of HRPPPs. In this framework, HRPPPs include, but are not limited to, programs that use the traditional IRB model. The complexity of significant and delicate issues that are encompassed in such a task merits an in-depth examination by IOM, and thus, the task is to be conducted in two phases.

This report represents the results of phase 1 of the IOM study. It examines the potential benefits and strengths that an accreditation strategy, such as those under development within the research community and at the direction of the VA (see Appendixes B and C), could bring to ongoing efforts to enhance HRPPPs. More specifically, the report addresses the following three tasks:

1. review and consider proposed human research review program[3] performance standards;

2. recommend standards for accreditation of HRPPPs, considering measures of structure, process, and performance, as well as resource sufficiency; and

---

[3] In the course of committee deliberations, the term "human research participant protection program" was substituted for "human research review program," as the former term better reflected the system of oversight that the committee hopes will result from its recommendations.

**3. recommend steps that the organizations and institutions that con-
duct research and that the federal government should take to collect and
analyze data to monitor and evaluate how well the system for protecting
human research participants is operating.**

This report therefore provides recommendations for core standards with
which to initiate pilot accreditation programs for HRPPPs, specific comments on
standards under development, and suggested interim actions that can be used to
initiate and monitor the impact of accreditation on the system and its ability to
achieve the intended goals. The recommendations, listed below, appear in Box 1,
at the conclusion of the Executive Summary, according to how they relate to the
three broad categories; that is, whether they respond to the goal of developing an
accreditation program, standards, or a system of evaluation. However, all comments are made in the context of the current policy and existing regulatory structures and without the benefit of a full examination of the underlying issues and
possible solutions.

The structures and processes constituting an accreditation system are only
coming into being and still need to be tested. Therefore, the committee's recommendations are aimed at a moving target. Its recommendations about accreditation standards in particular presume that those standards will evolve substantially, especially with the benefit of feedback from initial pilot tests. The
committee recommends standards for pilot testing of accreditation programs, but
the committee did not itself formulate those standards. It neither could nor
should have done so, for several reasons. First, the accreditation standards
should be formulated in a "bootstrap" process, with strong feedback between the
formulation of standards and direct experience with the implementation of
HRPPP standards. Second, accreditation bodies should be accountable for their
standards as well as their accreditation processes. Reliance on "IOM standards"
would thus undermine this alignment between authority and responsibility for
standard setting at a critical point in the development of (an) accreditation pro-
gram(s). Finally, the standards will evolve over time and will do so rapidly during initial pilot testing. This iterative process would not be possible with a set of
IOM standards produced at this time. As the committee formulated its recommendations, no pilot testing had taken place, and reliance on standards in advance of and independent of such testing runs contrary to early experience with
the development of new oversight mechanisms in general and past models of
accreditation in particular.

MAJOR FINDINGS

In accordance with its task, the committee reviewed available draft accreditation standards at the time of its deliberations. For this purpose, materials
developed by Public Responsibility in Medicine and Research (PRIM&R) and,

subsequently, the National Committee for Quality Assurance (NCQA), were provided to the committee. To assess those materials, the committee found it useful to use the following general criteria: (1) their scope and focus; (2) their relationship to the existing regulatory standards; and (3) the extent to which the standards can be consistently implemented, measured, and enforced, as well as their inclusion of various key elements. For more discussion on the review and elements considered, please see Chapter 3.

> **Finding 1:** The standards proposed by NCQA for VA facilities appear promising for use in the accreditation of VA facilities. Those same standards are the strongest basis for use in the accreditation of other research institutions (see Table 1). The committee regards the standards prepared by NCQA to be more suitable than those prepared by PRIM&R for not only pilot testing in VA facilities but also, with modification, for the accreditation of other research institutions.

> **Finding 2:** Neither set of proposed standards applies readily to the full range of research involving human participants or to the diversity of research institutions that conduct it. Both sets of standards understandably and reasonably start from the kinds of research and the types of research organizations where recent problems have been best documented. It is not clear, however, how standards should be applied to nonbiomedical research settings, contract management organizations, clinical trials cooperative groups, independent IRBs, central IRBs, site management organizations, or units of research sponsors that conduct human research (e.g., research units within federal agencies and private pharmaceutical, biotechnology, and device companies).

How the proposed standards can be adapted to the large and growing fraction of research not conducted in the framework of biomedical research institutions will be an important question to be addressed in pilot tests. This is problematic in two respects. First, many institutions performing research with humans are not primarily focused on clinical research, yet the standards have clearly been formulated with medical research in mind. Second, the accreditation system must cover all types of research organizations. A very large fraction, probably a majority, of clinical research is privately sponsored and conducted outside traditional medical research institutions for which both sets of standards were developed. Failure to include privately sponsored research reviewed by independent IRBs would not only exclude a significant fraction of research with humans but would also call into question whether the accreditation process was skewed in favor of academic health centers. It is premature to judge how accreditation can work for these organizations, but it is critical to include them in any credible accreditation system.

TABLE 1 Comparison of Draft NCQA and PRIM&R Accreditation Standards

Organization preparing standards	Strengths	Weaknesses
NCQA	• Direct linkage to quality improvement programs • Grounded in baseline regulatory requirements • Measurement criteria and data sources specified • Interpretive guidance provided • Accreditation process specified • IRB decision appeals process specified • Thresholds for compliance specified • Formulation of standards and accreditation of VA facilities by the same organization	• Because of an exclusive focus on VA facilities, will need to be modified for use for organizations for which standards were not originally designed[a] • Insufficient standards relating to participant involvement beyond informed consent • Insufficient attention to role of HRPPP accreditation vis-à-vis external research sponsors • Insufficient standards for research monitoring • Uncertain application to nonmedical research
PRIM&R	• Grounded in ethical principles of The Belmont Report[b] • Reflect strong expertise about IRB operations in academic health centers • Differentiate substandards for IRBs, institutions, and investigators	• Lack of specificity in standards for investigator and institutional obligations • Documentation standards for IRB record-keeping inapplicable to many IRBs • Uncertain application to nonmedical research, independent IRBs, contract research organizations, clinical trials cooperative groups, central IRBs, and other research organizations • Lack of cross-tabulation of standards to regulations

- Inadequate specification of data sources, except documentation standards

- Insufficient attention to role of HRPPP accreditation vis-à-vis external research sponsors

- Insufficient standards relating to participant involvement beyond informed consent

- Insufficient standards for research monitoring

- Lack of specificity regarding measures and thresholds for compliance

- Lack of interpretive guidance

- Lack of specificity regarding accreditation judgments

- Formulated with an inadequate link between responsibility for developing standards (an ongoing process) and responsibility for implementing accreditation process

---

[a] Although it is identified as a weakness in this table, the NCQA standards were designed only for VA facilities, so a lack of more general applicability is not a criticism of the NCQA formulation but is an observation about their use of the NCQA standards for purposes that the committee recommends, that is, for non-VA organizations.
[b] National Commission for the Protection of Human Subjects of Biomedical and Behavioral Research (1979).

In the course of the second, more comprehensive, phase of the committee's work, the committee may or may not revisit HRPPP accreditation. The future report will certainly address other strategies for improvement to supplement this report, such as educating investigators, augmenting resources for research oversight (at both the federal and the local levels), enhancing oversight of ongoing research (including monitoring bodies and reporting mechanisms), and other strategies.

RECOMMENDATIONS

Recommendation 1: Pursue Accreditation Through Pilot Testing as One Approach

Accreditation of HRPPPs should be pursued as *one* promising approach to improving the human participant protection system. The first step is implementation of pilot programs to test standards, establish accreditation processes, and build confidence in accreditation organizations. This effort should be evaluated for its impact on protecting the rights and interests of participants in 3 to 5 years.

The process of establishing an accreditation system typically takes many years, and it must be continually adjusted, particularly in its initial phases. Current efforts to establish accreditation systems are just under way, and the proposed standards are new and untested. The process for the accreditation of HRPPPs is still being configured, and the organizaitons thus far identified to carry it out are taking on an unprecedented task. Two specific approaches have been presented to the committee. The process that is furthest along is a nascent accrediation process for the VA medical facilities being conducted by NCQA under a contract with the VA. That contract commenced in May 2000. Another organization, the Association for the Accreditation of Human Research Protection Programs (AAHRPP), was originally incorporated in March 2000, but its formal establishment is still under way (see Chapter 2).

These emerging accreditation programs are best viewed as pilot projects that will have to be evaluated in light of experience. Any accreditation system must be constructed as an evolving tool and part of a long-term strategy and cannot be expected to immediately correct deficiencies in the HRPPP system. As a component of a long-term strategy to improve the quality of research oversight, however, a nongovernmental accreditation process has promise and should be tested as soon as possible. The logical first step is to continue the VA accreditation program. The second step is to pilot test accreditation in academic health centers and private research organizations whose HRPPPs conform to the organizational structures for which both sets of draft standards were formulated: those that conduct research, directly employ investigators, and have IRBs. The

NCQA standards appear to be closer to adaptation for such use than the PRIM&R standards do (see Recommendation 9).

Recommendation 2: Establish a Nongovernmental Accreditation Organization(s)

Organizations formulating accreditation standards and carrying out the accreditation process should be independent, nongovernmental organizations. These organizations should include within their programmatic leaderships the perspectives of the relevant stakeholders in the applicant HRPPP community (i.e., institutions, investigators, sponsors, and participants).

An accreditation process is only as credible as the organizations that carry it out. The foremost criterion is independence (Hamm, 1997). Organizations formulating standards and conducting the accreditation process should

1. be national in scope;
2. be familiar with the operations of institutions that apply for accreditation; and
3. incorporate the perspectives of research participants within their programmatic leadership.

An accreditation process should directly involve the kinds of institutions being accredited, but an accreditation organization should not be beholden to any particular stakeholder or interest group. Accreditation bodies for HRPPPs will require input from academic health centers, organizations representing research sponsors, nongovernmental research organizations, private firms developing products and services tested in studies with humans, participants, IRB members and staff from both academic and nonacademic institutions, research administrators in both academic and nonacademic institutions, and individuals from a range of research fields appropriate to the intended range of applicant institutions.

Research participant representatives will be particularly important in formulating the overall goals of the HRPPP systems, and their perspectives should be systematically solicited in both the formulation of standards and the execution of the accreditation process. This involvement will also include representation on groups that set standards and teams that conduct external evaluations and site visits. National accreditation bodies should seek to involve organizations that have both a genuine national constituency that corresponds to the interests of the research participants[4] and a demonstrated familiarity with the research process and research protection rules and regulations (see Recommendation 8).

---

[4] In the case of the VA, for example, this would include national veterans organizations; for medical research, this would include health advocacy organizations; and for community-based or population-based research, this would include organizations representing the communities or the full range of subpopulations sampled.

Recommendation 3: Articulate Sound Goals Within Accreditation Standards

The goals of accreditation standards should be to ensure
1. That the proposed research promises to contribute knowledge sufficient to justify research involving human participants;
2. independent review of research by a board knowledgeable about protection standards and the fields of research being reviewed;
3. that the perspectives of participants are represented on IRBs, on research monitoring bodies, and throughout the research oversight system;
4. that IRB members do not review protocols with which they have financial or nonfinancial conflicts of interest;[5]
5. that investigator and institutional conflicts of interest, both financial and nonfinancial, are disclosed to IRBs and participants and are managed responsibly by research institutions;
6. a review process that balances risks and potential benefits, keeps risks to the minimum necessary, and monitors research on a continuing basis;
7. that an effective process for obtaining voluntary informed consent of participants is in place;
8. that policies and procedures are in place to assess the quality of HRPPP operations, enhance accountability, and improve performance;
9. there is fairness in recruitment and selection of participants;
10. that the privacy and confidentiality of research participants are protected; and
11. that the HRPPP is transparent so that participants can judge the research process to be trustworthy.

Recommendation 4: Establish Flexible, Ethics-Based, and Meaningful Standards

Accreditation standards should meet the following minimal criteria:
1. They should be based on sound and widely accepted ethical principles.[6]

---

[5] The committee does not mean that any member who could have a conflict with any conceivable protocol coming to an IRB for review should be excluded from service on an IRB but, rather, means that the individual should recuse himself or herself from reviewing such protocols.

6. They should be flexible and adapted to different kinds of research and different research institutions.

7. They should encourage accredited organizations to shift from a culture that relies on external compliance checks to a culture that puts safety and voluntary participation foremost.

8. They should facilitate compliance with federal regulations but should aim to move an organization toward having stronger protection of human research participants.

9. To the extent possible, they should focus on the use of meaningful measures of how well the rights and interests of research participants are being protected rather than simple determination of whether informed-consent statements have been signed or IRB meetings were duly constituted.

The committee believes that the draft NCQA standards are close to meeting the criteria in Recommendations 3 and 4 for pilot testing in VA facilities, and if they are modified as suggested under Recommendation 9, they could be used as the basis for pilot tests of HRPPP standards outside VA facilities.

Recommendation 5: Accommodate Distinct Research Methods and Models Within Accreditation Programs

The accreditation process should accommodate other research organizations in addition to the traditional models provided by academic health centers and VA facilities. The accreditation process should also cover research other than clinical research.

Proposed NCQA standards were designed for VA facilities only. PRIM&R standards were prepared with a broader range of institutions in mind, but the committee heard strong, consistent comments that they do not fully recognize either the diversity of institutions or the full range of research (IOM, 2001). The standards proposed by NCQA and PRIM&R focus on HRPPPs that comprise a research institution, investigators, and IRBs. These elements are present in VA

---

[6] The principles laid out in *The Belmont Report* are one foundation (National Commission for the Protection of Human Subjects of Biomedical and Behavioral Research, 1979). Accreditation standards, however, should also incorporate the recommendations of the President's Commission for the Study of Ethical Problems in Medicine and Biomedical and Behavioral Research (President's Commission, 1981, 1983), the recommendations of the Advisory Committee for Human Radiation Experiments (ACHRE, 1995), recommendations presented in reports of the National Bioethics Advisory Commission (NBAC, 1998, 1999a,b, forthcoming-a, forthcoming-b), the recommendations of the Office of the Inspector General of DHHS (DHHS OIG, 1998b, 2000b), and the recommendations of the General Accounting Office (GAO, 1996). In addition, recommendations from reports and declarations of private bodies and independent scholars should be incorporated. This presupposes that an advisory apparatus is available to cull this literature.

facilities, academic health centers, and some other research organizations. Many organizations that might reasonably apply for HRPPP accreditation, however, do not conform to the traditional research organization model. Independent IRBs do not directly conduct research, for example, and so entire sections of the proposed standards are inapplicable to them.

To be credible, the accreditation process should expand to include independent IRBs; cooperative groups; contract research organizations; site management organizations; units within federal research agencies that conduct their own research; and units of pharmaceutical, medical device, and biotechnology firms that carry out research with human participants. The accreditation process must be sufficiently elastic to accommodate all major organizational structures involved in research with humans. Failure to cover the full range of research organizations under an accreditation program would undermine the credibility of the accreditation process so essential to the program's success in two ways. First, it would eliminate a large and growing fraction of research with humans, and second, it could be perceived as a subterfuge to protect the competitive advantage of academic health centers to the detriment of private independent IRBs on the basis of categorical exclusion rather than quality. Yet, neither NCQA nor PRIM&R draft standards can be directly applied to many organizations conducting research with humans. Discovering how to do this with one or several sets of standards, whether under one accreditation body or a few, will be an important question to address in pilot tests.

Accreditation of an independent IRB, for example, might use only the subset of standards pertinent to IRBs, but doing so would also require assurance regarding the functions covered by proposed standards that pertain to investigators, research institutions, and research participants, as well as standards not yet incorporated into NCQA or PRIM&R standards (but covered by the guidelines of the International Conference on Harmonisation; see Chapter 3) pertaining to sponsors. Independent IRBs could be accredited with such assurances, perhaps on the basis of binding written agreements between the independent IRB and the research sponsors contracting for its services.

Another approach would be to accredit the organization that does directly control all the relevant elements of an HRPPP (e.g., a contract research organization that has a formal agreement with an independent IRB to review all its protocols, the research unit of a private firm, the unit of a federal agency that performs research, or a clinical trials cooperative group). These approaches are not mutually exclusive, but neither approach is reflected in the NCQA and PRIM&R draft standards. One of the virtues of a nongovernmental voluntary accreditation process is its flexibility, and nongovernmental accreditation bodies should not find it difficult to accommodate disparate organizational structures, but it is not yet clear how the current proposed standards or accreditation processes would do so.

How to apply the proposed standards to nonmedical research institutions[7] is also controversial and should be explicitly addressed in pilot accreditation programs. Commentary at the committee's January 2001 public forum stressed that proposed HRPPP standards focus almost entirely on clinical research. Although the proposed PRIM&R standards include many that would be used only "if applicable" to a given applicant organization, a set of standards developed for the social and behavioral sciences or for population-based studies *ab initio* would not include many of the "if applicable" standards and would expand or rephrase other standards.

The committee believes that the same principles for protection of the rights and interests of research participants apply to all research, and in that sense the same general standard of conduct should prevail. It is an open question, however, whether the best accreditation strategy would be to use one set of operational standards for all research. That might well prove viable, but it also might prove better to encourage the evolution of different specific standards for different kinds of research institutions. Those in the best position to judge this will be organizations devising the accreditation processes, not this committee or the federal government. Whether to develop one set of standards or a few sets of standards specific to a few different classes of research organizations should not be decided by fiat but should be decided in light of experience gained through pilot accreditation programs that include medical and nonmedical sites.

Accreditation demonstration programs can begin by focusing on the research institutions for which they were designed, but they might evolve in many different ways. In the future, there could be one or a few accreditation bodies and one or a few sets of accreditation standards, and many different kinds of organizations will continue to be involved in research with human participants.

Recommendation 6: Base Standards on Existing Regulations

Accreditation standards should start from federal regulations for the protection of human research participants but should augment those regulations. The process should be iterative and continual, with evolution of both accreditation standards and the operations of accredited organizations, creating incentives for accredited organizations to improve.

---

[7] By "nonmedical institutions," the committee refers to organizations that conduct or review research that is not primarily clinical. Some research institutions, for example, concentrate on national surveys or demographic research; others mainly review student research projects. Entire research centers are devoted to epidemiology, population and community-based research, or public health. Some academic and independent private research institutes focus on studies in anthropology, oral history, sociology, psychology, journalism, law, and political science. These fields have widely different norms and methods, and the nature of the risks for participants also differs.

Accreditation standards start from a base of regulations governing research with humans. The regulations, in turn, are based on a set of principles for the ethical conduct of research (see Recommendation 4). The standards proposed by NCQA are tightly coupled to the existing federal regulations, but they also incorporate quality improvement processes that could evolve into a different set of standards over time. The NCQA strategy will therefore focus first on facilitating compliance with existing regulations but, importantly, will provide a means to raise the quality of protection standards over time. By using standards that emphasize processes of continual quality improvement instead of an exclusive focus on regulatory compliance, the way may be open to the development of future standards that center on HRPPP performance, in addition to the current focus on documentation. For example, an HRPPP that demonstrates that it can ensure informed consent because it has data showing that participants understand the protocols in which they are enrolled could begin to supplant or augment paper audits of signed informed-consent forms. This strategy therefore has the potential to introduce the desired flexibility and focus on outcomes into the oversight system.

Accreditation will not be successful until it is widely accepted as a mark of excellence. It should also serve as an educational tool to raise the median overall performance. To do this, accreditation standards and the processes in which they will be used must incorporate consistent feedback from the parties involved in the various aspects of an HRPPP. Those who encounter problems in the research system—participants or people who care about them, investigators submitting research for review by an IRB, institutions negotiating agreements to perform sponsored research, anyone who notices something going awry in the course of a study, or data safety and monitoring boards that note a pattern in reported adverse events—need simple, consistent ways to bring their concerns to light. In addition, they need ways to bring relevant information into the procedure for the review of the process, including the functioning of both the HRPPP system and the accreditation process.

One of the chief advantages of a voluntary nongovernmental accreditation system over a mandatory government process is that it can evolve over time without requiring new federal regulations at each step. It took 10 years for 18 agencies to adopt the federal Common Rule governing human research (45 CFR 46, Subpart A), and at least 3 agencies that conduct human research remain outside of the rule.[8] The current regulatory system is demonstrably unresponsive to dramatic changes in how research is conducted; a nongovernmental accreditation

---

[8] OPRR noted three agencies that appeared to sponsor research with human participants but that were not signatories to the Common Rule: the National Endowment for the Humanities, the U.S. Department of Labor, and the Nuclear Regulatory Commission, as cited in a draft report forthcoming from the National Bioethics Advisory Committee (NBAC, forthcoming-b).

system may be more responsive by comparison and would comport with Circular No. A-119 of the Office of Management and Budget, which urges the use of nongovernmental "voluntary consensus standards" where possible (OMB, 1998).[9]

The committee envisions an accreditation process that will continually evolve, updating standards over time. The operations of organizations seeking accreditation will also evolve. The parallel evolution of accreditation standards and HRPPP operations should be an iterative process, with the formulation of standards efficiently informed by knowledge acquired in the accreditation process. The formulation of standards, the conduct of accreditation site visits, and external evaluation must therefore be intimately linked.

Recommendation 7: Incorporate Continuous Quality Improvement Mechanisms into Standards

Accreditation organizations should emphasize the process of self-study, evaluation, and continual quality improvement among applicants. They should move beyond documentation of informed consent and protocol review, which, although essential, do not of themselves protect the rights and interests of research participants.

Standards should aim to improve outcomes and should not overly prescribe how to achieve the specified objectives. Rather, they should focus on the core standards that apply across programs and that are essential to a quality HRPPP. Current proposed standards generally reinforce the documentation practices required by federal regulations but do not go beyond these regulatory requirements. In general, both entities seeking accreditation and accreditation bodies should identify exemplary performance and best practices, providing benchmarks for the research community at large and making information on organization performance openly available to the public and policy makers.

Linkage to quality improvement strategies also offers a path to achievements well beyond regulatory compliance. For example, an HRPPP demonstrating a particularly reliable system for the monitoring of participant safety or the reporting of problems in ongoing research could have a competitive advantage over nonaccredited competitors in seeking support from sponsors or having access to participants, researchers, or students. The committee concurs with this strategy which was incorporated into the standards proposed by NCQA and recommends that it should also be applied to non-VA research organizations.

---

[9] Circular No. A-119 was intended mainly for technical standards pertaining to products, but it also contemplates "related management systems practices."

Recommendation 8: Directly Involve Research Participants in Accreditation Programs and HRPPPs

The formulation of accreditation standards, the accreditation process, and HRPPP operations should directly involve research participants.[10]

Accreditation bodies should formally solicit input from and directly involve the groups of people who will be studied in research carried out by the organizations that they will accredit. Participant perspectives are an essential element in research design, especially as it pertains to informed consent and the minimization of risk, and participant representatives should be directly involved in IRB review and should be members of the programmatic leaderships of accreditation review groups, site visit teams, monitoring boards, and oversight and advisory groups in research institutions. Standards should also reflect stronger participant involvement beyond securing signatures on informed-consent documents.

Recommendation 9: Use Modified NCQA Standards to Initiate Pilot Programs

Pilot accreditation programs should start from the accreditation standards and processes proposed by NCQA for VA facilities, as adapted for use in other organizational contexts. In expanding the draft NCQA accreditation standards for use beyond VA facilities, the standards should be strengthened in six specific ways as pilot testing commences.

The PRIM&R standards were prepared for a broad set of potential applicant organizations, which would include but not be restricted to academic health centers. The NCQA standards were explicitly prepared for accreditation of VA medical facilities. In this instance, the applicant pool is defined, and, in fact, pilot tests that will use those standards are being planned as this report goes to press.

As noted throughout this discussion of report recommendations, the committee regards the NCQA standards as an excellent starting point for accreditation of VA facilities. The committee recommends, however, that the NCQA standards be strengthened in six areas, discussed in more detail in Chapter 3, to specify (1) how investigators will be reviewed beyond the review of the protocols that they submit for IRB approval; (2) whether and how research sponsors will be assessed in the accreditation process; (3) how participants will be involved in setting standards and accrediting HRPPPs; (4) how oversight mecha-

---

[10] By "participants," the committee refers to those whose background and expertise are credible to a lay constituency external to the research institution and who are knowledgeable about the research process and research protections. The term is further defined in Chapter 1.

nisms can ensure participants' safety in ongoing research; (5) the steps that research institutions and their leadership can take to cultivate a culture that puts the safety and interests of research participants foremost; and (6) mechanisms by which research institutions and, where applicable, research sponsors can be held accountable for ensuring sufficient funding, structural support, and professional rewards for HRPPPs.

The NCQA standards, if improved as recommended, could also be used—by NCQA, AAHRPP, or other accreditation organizations—as the basis for the development of accreditation standards for non-VA research organizations.

Recommendation 10: Begin Collecting Data and Assessing Impacts of Accreditation Now

DHHS should commission studies to gather baseline data on the current system of protections for human participants in the research that it oversees and to assess whether the system is improving over time.

Baseline data are needed on the following:

- a taxonomy of research institutions: the number of institutions conducting research with human participants and the number of studies of different types (e.g., clinical trials, surveys, student projects, and behavioral studies) approved by their HRPPPs;
- a taxonomy of IRBs: the number of IRBs and what fraction of them are primarily devoted to studies of particular types;
- a taxonomy of studies with humans: the number and distribution of investigations with humans under way by type of study, for example, clinical trials of various stages, observational studies, cross-sectional and longitudinal surveys, and social science experiments;
- the number of people involved in research and, among them, how many are involved in research with more than minimal risk;
- the fraction of studies with more than minimal risk that have formal safety monitoring boards and how (and how well) those boards operate;
- the type and number of inquiries, investigations, and sanctions by FDA and the Office for Human Research Protections; and
- the type and number of serious or unanticipated adverse events attributable to research.

DHHS should also commission studies of how the databases for existing clinical trials and other research resources could be used to assess how well the system of research protections is operating and, specifically, whether accreditation is having measurable impacts (e.g., by comparing accredited and nonaccredited institutions or by comparing institutions before and after accreditation).

Other studies are needed to bolster the nascent literature on how well research participants understand the studies that they join, which risks matter most to them, and what forms of informed consent are most effective. Several new initiatives to enhance clinical research in particular are under way, and the National Institutes of Health has initiated new programs to improve research monitoring. DHHS should evaluate these efforts not only for their primary purpose of improving clinical research but also for how they can improve HRPPPs.

Recommendation 11: Initiate Federal Studies Evaluating Accreditation

The U.S. Congress should request an evaluation of accreditation pilot programs from the General Accounting Office. The Secretary of Health and Human Services should consider requesting a parallel evaluation from the Office of the Inspector General of DHHS.

An evaluation process that is independent of AAHRPP, NCQA, and other accreditation bodies can help policy makers decide on the value of accreditation as an improvement strategy several years hence. Without such an evaluation, Congress and the executive branch will be positioned little better than they are today to make prudent choices about how to improve HRPPPs in 5 years. Research pursued under Recommendation 10 can provide some baseline information, but it cannot substitute for a thorough evaluation of the accreditation pilot projects themselves. Furthermore, the evaluation efforts would benefit in several respects if they were initiated soon, while the pilot projects are getting under way. Evaluators could observe which organizations seek accreditation and which ones do not. They could also conduct interviews with organization officials who are making a particular choice to find out why and what they perceive the benefits or problems of HRPPP accreditation programs to be. If multiple accreditation bodies emerge, the evaluation should compare their effectiveness.

The HRPPP accreditation process should be evaluated not only according to whether it has improved protections for human research participants but also according to whether resources devoted to accreditation could be spent to equal or better effect on other ways to improve HRPPP oversight such as education, research monitoring, and improved feedback mechanisms. Evaluation should take into account both the costs of establishing a national accreditation system and the costs to applicant organizations. The costs to applicant organizations will include direct costs for the accreditation process and also costs for the preparation for and following up on the accreditation process.

CONCLUDING REMARKS

In summary, the committee has addressed through its recommendations what it believes are the fundamental components necessary to initiate and effectively utilize an accreditation process and a set of accreditation standards to enhance participant protection in human research. Box 1 presents the committee's recommendations according to the three phases intrinsic to the implementation of an accreditation process: development of the program, development of standards, and evaluating the program.

First, to develop the accreditation program, accreditation of HRPPPs should be pursued through pilot programs as one method to enhance the overall protection of participants taking part in research. This effort should be led by nongovernmental accreditation bodies with both the responsibility and the authority to craft and implement accreditation standards. Maintenance of these tasks within one or a few independent entities allows data collection and the experience gained through the process of accreditation to be tethered tightly to the timely evolution of standards. Further, any accreditation standards must encompass an assessment of participant involvement in local research oversight, greater specificity about the responsibilities of research sponsors, and integration of research monitoring, professional education, and quality improvement into the oversight system.

Second, with respect to the development of accreditation standards, the committee believes that the NCQA draft standards should be adopted as a starting point. They will, however, require modification to include the components in Recommendation 9 and to accommodate disparate research environments and disciplines. This recommendation stems from the NCQA standard's explicit underpinning in federal regulations, their reliance upon rigorous quality improvement programs, and the resulting potential to move from a system overly focused on administrative compliance to one that emphasizes flexibility in achieving protection of participants in research.

Finally, efforts to evaluate the ability of accreditation programs to improve HRPPP function (i.e., ensure participant protection) should begin now. The committee suggests two complementary strategies: 1) data collection to assess systemic improvement over time; and 2) independent, comprehensive analysis of the effectiveness and relative cost of accreditation programs in achieving desired outcomes.

These recommendations are intended to guide the federal government and research entities in their immediate efforts to ensure that high-quality, innovative research never sacrifices the rights and safety of those individuals who voluntarily assume the risks inherent in research with humans.

BOX 1 Summary of Committee's Recommendations According to the Three Implementation Phases of an Accreditation Process

Development of an Accreditation Program:

Pursue Accreditation Through Pilot Testing as One Approach
    (Recommendation 1)
Establish (a) Nongovernmental Accreditation Organization(s)
    (Recommendation 2)
Accommodate Distinct Research Methods and Models Within Accreditation Programs
    (Recommendation 5)
Directly Involve Research Participants in Accreditation Programs & HRPPPs
    (Recommendation 8)

Development of Standards:

Articulate Sound Goals Within Accreditation Standards
    (Recommendation 3)
Establish Flexible, Ethics-Based, and Meaningful Standards
    (Recommendation 4)
Base Standards on Existing Regulations
    (Recommendation 6)
Incorporate Continuous Quality Improvement Mechanisms into Standards
    (Recommendation 7)
Use Modified NCQA Standards to Initiate Pilot Programs
    (Recommendation 9)

Development of an Evaluation Process:

Begin Collecting Data and Assessing Impacts of Accreditation Now
    (Recommendation 10)
Initiate Federal Studies Evaluating Accreditation
    (Recommendation 11)

1

Introduction, Background, and Definitions

Proper preparations should be made and adequate facilities provided to pro-tect the experimental subject against even remote possibilities of injury, dis-ability, or death.

Principle 7, the Nuremberg Code

The protection of individuals who volunteer to participate in research is es-sential to the ethical conduct of research. Such protections were not explicitly and systematically addressed in the United States, however, until the late 1940s, when scientists and policy makers recognized the need to respond to crimes committed by Nazi scientists during World War II. Since then national and in-ternational policies have evolved to create a system of protections requiring the involvement of investigators, research sponsors, research institutions, health care providers, federal agencies, and patient and consumer groups. This evolu-tion is worth tracking to appreciate what brings this report to the forefront at this time; that is, how can this complex system of protections be assessed in a reli-able and valid way to ensure that it is effective, efficient, and accountable—that "proper preparations" have been made and that "adequate facilities" have been provided to protect the experimental subjects of research?

ORGANIZATION OF THE REPORT

Before beginning the discussion leading to the recommendations contained within this report, the committee notes that this document focuses narrowly on

23

the accreditation of programs that are charged with the responsibility of protecting individuals who volunteer for research. This first chapter provides the relevant background preceding this work, as well as discussion pertaining to the committee's concept of a human research participant protection program (HRPPP) and related terminology. Chapter 2 explores various models of accreditation. It also focuses on how accreditation might apply to activities surrounding protection of human research participants and explores the process for such a system.

Chapter 3 centers on the issue of standards; that is, what values and measurements should be used to address an organization's level of performance and expectations for activities that affect the protection of participants in human research? In response to its charge, the committee reviewed the draft Public Responsibility in Medicine and Research (PRIM&R) standards and those developed by the National Committee for Quality Assurance (NCQA). Chapter 3 presents the committee's recommendations about standards for accreditation.

Chapter 4 focuses on issues in evaluating and analyzing a system of accreditation. In response to the committee's third task, this chapter includes committee recommendations for steps that the federal government should take to collect and analyze data that can be used to monitor and evaluate how well the system for protecting human research participants is operating.

A SHORT HISTORY OF HUMAN SUBJECTS PROTECTIONS IN THE UNITED STATES

In response to the atrocities committed by Nazi scientists during World War II, the Nuremberg Military Tribunal created the Nuremberg Code, a set of 10 principles for research involving human participants, including an absolute requirement for voluntary consent (Nuremburg Code, 1946–1949; *United States v. Karl Brandt et al.* The Medical Case 1946–1949). The Nuremberg principles placed primary responsibility on the investigator to ensure that research was ethically conducted. At the same time that the Nuremberg Trial was proceeding, anticipating the need for a rapid response to concerns about research abuses, the American Medical Association adopted its first code of research ethics for physicians in 1946, outlining principles to be followed in conducting research with human subjects (AMA Judicial Council, 1946).

Over the ensuing two decades, U.S. policy in this area evolved, addressing prohibitions on research involving vulnerable or special populations and eventually requiring independent review of research and written consent for "hazardous" research (ACHRE, 1995). The Kefauver-Harris Amendments to the Federal Food, Drug, and Cosmetic Act required the Food and Drug Administration (FDA) to evaluate new drugs for safety as well as efficacy, significantly expanding the power of the federal government to influence the conduct of clinical trials in particular.[1] One of the provisions of this act required the informed consent of participants in the testing of new drugs. The federal policies were slowly moving away from reliance on the investigator as the sole focus of decision making about ethical research and more toward a policy that required independent review of research and retrieval of voluntary informed consent. This meant that the responsibility, although still on the investigator, was also being placed on the institutions that support and conduct research.

By the 1960s, however, few research institutions had in place a system for protecting research subjects, despite requests by the National Institutes of Health (NIH) that they do so (Faden and Beauchamp, 1986). A 1966 U.S. Public Health Service (PHS) policy required independent review of research by a committee of the investigator's "institutional associates" (PHS, 1966). Later, NIH would create the Office for Protection from Research Risks (OPRR) and take the lead in the protection of research subjects in research conducted or sponsored by the U.S. Department of Health and Human Services (DHHS).

The need for enhanced efforts to protect research subjects was underlined in 1966 when Henry Beecher published an article presenting 22 examples of "unethical or questionably ethical studies" that had appeared in mainstream medical journals (Beecher, 1966). One of these studies involved injection of the hepatitis virus into children seeking admission to the Willowbrook State School for the Retarded in New York. Although parental consent was obtained, it was likely uninformed and certainly suspect because of undue influence, that is, concerns of parents that their children could not be enrolled in the school if they refused to participate (ACHRE, 1995). Then, in 1972, details emerged about the Tuskegee Syphilis Study, begun in the 1930s (Heller, 1972). The study attempted to trace over several decades the natural history of syphilis in poor, African-American males living in Alabama. Not only were the participants not told the purpose of the study, but they were also led to believe that they were receiving treatment (Gamble, 1997; Heller, 1972; Jones, 1981). PHS deemed the study unethical and stopped it, offering the surviving participants antibiotic treatment.

A PHS advisory panel reviewing the Tuskegee study determined that existing procedures for the protection of research subjects were inadequate and that the U.S. Congress should establish a "permanent body with the authority to regulate *at least* all federally supported research involving human subjects" (Tuskegee Syphilis Study Ad Hoc Advisory Panel, 1973, p. 23). Subsequent congressional hearings led to passage of the National Research Act, which established the National Commission for the Protection of Human Subjects of Biomedical and Behavioral Research (the National Commission) to provide analyses of the ethics and policies related to the conduct of research with human subjects.[2]

---

[1] Federal Food, Drug, and Cosmetic Act of 1938. P.L. 75-717, 52, Stat. 1040, as amended 21 U.S.C. 31 et seq.

[2] National Research Act of 1974. P.L. 93-348 (1974).

In 1979, the National Commission published *The Belmont Report*, which identifies three basic principles for the ethical conduct of research with human subjects: respect for persons, beneficence, and justice. In response to this report, DHHS and FDA revised their regulations, creating in 1981 the Federal Policy for the Protection of Human Subjects in Research.[3] The National Commission described the then-emergent structure and function of ethics review boards at research institutions, which later became known as institutional review boards (IRBs). IRBs became the roof beam in the framework for the protection of the rights and interests of human participants in research and remain so today.

In 1981, the President's Commission for the Study of Ethical Problems in Medicine and Biomedical and Behavioral Research (the President's Commission) was established. Two of its reports focused on the system of protection of human participants in research (President's Commission, 1981, 1983). In *Implementing Human Research Regulations*, the President's Commission recommended that, "There should be a uniform Federal system documenting the implementation of the regulations through prior assurance and periodic site visits" (President's Commission, 1983, p. 3).

Eventually, the federal government would attempt to standardize the human subjects regulations across agencies and departments. In 1991, the regulations, now known as the "Common Rule" (Subpart A, 45 CFR 46), were simultaneously published in the *Federal Register* by 15 departments and agencies. By 2001, 18 agencies have adopted the Common Rule, and numerous additional international documents and guidelines have been developed and revised (see Box 1-1). The regulations used across the federal government prescribe requirements for research involving human subjects, including the functions, operations, and compositions of IRBs; IRB review of research; record keeping; and requirements for informed consent.

MORE RECENT EVENTS

Advisory Committee on Human Radiation Experiments

In 1993, the nation was shocked by a series of news articles in the *Albuquerque Tribune* that revealed experiments involving injection of plutonium into humans. This touched off national press coverage and subsequent revelations about Cold War-era radiation experiments conducted with civilian and military populations. In response, President Bill Clinton established the Advisory Committee on Human Radiation Experiments (ACHRE) to investigate reports of federally sponsored human research involving radioactive materials conducted

---

[3] 45 CFR 46; the FDA regulations are at 21 CFR 50, 56.

BOX 1-1 Relevant International Codes

Research is a global enterprise. U.S. commissions have built on and worked in parallel with codes developed elsewhere in the world, some of which also set a context for the present committee's work. Several international codes articulate principles for the ethical conduct of research. The **Declaration of Helsinki** is perhaps the best known among these. In its current form, the declaration contains 32 statements of principle to guide medical research. Its conceptual foundation is the medical ethics of the doctor-patient relationship, and this is extended to medical research via an investigator-subject relationship. The declaration opens with general statements of moral norms, the duties of physicians, and the subordinate role of science when it comes into conflict with the human rights of human subjects, followed by sections on research per se and research combined with medical care.

The **Council for International Organizations of Medical Sciences** (CIOMS) prepares the *International Ethical Guidelines for Biomedical Research Involving Human Subjects.* The first CIOMS guidelines were published in 1982, followed by revision in 1993, and they are again being revised, with public release expected in the next year (CIOMS, 1982, 1993).

The **International Conference on Harmonisation** has developed detailed guidelines specific to drug trials and for good clinical practice (International Conference on Harmonisation of Technical Requirements for Registration of Pharmaceuticals for Human Use, 1996, 1997) and many other guidelines on other aspects of testing of pharmaceutical products. The International Conference on Harmonisation was formed in 1990 and involves government agencies and pharmaceutical trade organizations from the European Union, Japan, and the United States (International Conference on Harmonisation, 1998). Its guidelines are not just for research that crosses national borders but, in fact, constitute guidance for trials of any size and are recognized formally by the Food and Drug Administration.

Several governments, including those of India and Canada, have prepared guidelines for research that are recognized by the U.S. Office of Human Research Protections (CECHR, Indian Council of Medical Research, 2000; NSERC, 2000; OHRP, 2000a). The **Indian Council of Medical Research** guidelines apply to biomedical research, and the **Tri-Council Statement** from Canada applies to research under the Natural Sciences and Engineering Council, the Social Sciences and Humanities Research Council, and the Institutes of Health Research.

between 1944 and 1972. ACHRE's work is a direct precedent to several current activities. As part of its charge, ACHRE also assessed the current state of protections for research subjects. In its final report, ACHRE concluded that it had found "evidence of serious deficiencies in some parts of the current system" (ACHRE, 1995, p. 797). In particular, ACHRE cited variability in the quality of IRBs, confusion on the part of research participants about whether they were to receive therapeutic benefit from volunteering for studies, and concern about the adequacy of the consent process. ACHRE urged that (1) federal oversight of human subject protections focus on outcomes and performance rather than paperwork reviews and intermittent audits for cause, (2) sanctions for violation be authorized and be in proportion to the seriousness of the violation, and (3) protections be extended to research that is not federally funded.

A study commissioned by NIH and published after release of the ACHRE report corroborated many of the ACHRE committee's findings. The study was based on a survey of IRBs and investigators at research institutions holding a federal assurance agreement with NIH. It found that an estimated half million people were involved in research under IRB-reviewed protocols and that the number of protocols had more than quadrupled in the two decades since the National Commission had last surveyed IRBs (Bell et al., 1998). That report concluded that the system of protection was by and large functioning adequately, but it did point to a mounting workload and the intermittent emergence of research scandals.

ACHRE also called for the creation of a national commission "to provide for the continuing interpretation and application of ethics rules and principles for the conduct of human subject research in an open and public forum" (ACHRE, 1995, p. 821). President Clinton's executive order creating the National Bioethics Advisory Commission (NBAC) implemented this recommendation.[4]

The National Bioethics Advisory Commission

NBAC was established by executive order in October 1995 and was asked by President Clinton to look into the protection of human subjects in research, with "protection of the rights and welfare of human research subjects" listed as its first priority (Clinton, 1995). As one of its first actions, in May 1997 NBAC unanimously resolved that "no person in the United States should be enrolled in research without the twin protections of informed consent by an authorized person and independent review of the risks and benefits of the research" (NBAC, forthcoming-b, p. 26). NBAC issued subsequent reports on research involving those with impaired decision-making capacity (NBAC, 1998), research using human biological materials (NBAC, 1999a), and ethical issues in human stem

---

[4] NBAC's establishment was also a culmination of long-standing interest in a bioethics commission among members of Congress, such as Senators Mark Hatfield and Edward Kennedy and Rep. Henry Waxman, as well as a 1993 congressional report and the President's Science Advisor, John H. Gibbons (OTA, U.S. Congress, 1993).

cell research (NBAC, 1999b), all of which address issues of research oversight and IRB function. Forthcoming reports will address ethical principles for U.S. interests conducting clinical trials abroad (NBAC, forthcoming-a) and describe a 5-year review of the adequacy of the system of human subjects protection in the United States (NBAC, forthcoming-b).

Reports from DHHS Office of the Inspector General

In June 1998, the Office of the Inspector General (OIG) of DHHS issued a report, *Institutional Review Boards: A Time for Reform* (DHHS OIG, 1998b). The report's foremost finding was that "the effectiveness of IRBs is in jeopardy" (p. ii) and that IRBs are facing overwhelming demands. A system that was originally devised as a volunteer effort to oversee a much smaller research effort in the 1970s was characterized as contending with its growing burden with scant resources. Recommendations included better training of IRB members and investigators, recasting of federal requirements to give IRBs more flexibility yet require more accountability, reduction of potential conflicts of interest among IRBs to enhance independence, and improvement of feedback to IRBs about developments in multisite trials and prior reviews of research plans. Echoing one of the charges to the present committee, the DHHS OIG report called for greater attention to the development and reading of indicators of how well IRBs were doing their job.

A Time for Reform was the flagship in a convoy of DHHS OIG reports on the protection of human research subjects. Three other DHHS OIG reports came out at the same time: (1) promising approaches to improving protections, (2) a description of the IRB process, and (3) a description of the emergence of independent boards, that is, IRBs that mainly review drug, device, and biologics trials sponsored by private industry under FDA regulations (DHHS OIG, 1998c,d,e). In April 2000, the DHHS OIG issued an update on *A Time for Reform*. It noted the increased enforcement efforts of both OPRR and FDA but little overall progress on its other recommendations (DHHS OIG, 2000b). DHHS OIG staff testified at hearings in both the U.S. House and U.S. Senate as Congress turned its attention to human subject protections in the year 2000 (Grob, 2000). The April 2000 DHHS OIG update specifically lauded the efforts of PRIM&R to develop standards for accreditation of IRBs and research institutions. A pair of reports published in June 2000 focused on recruiting human subjects, with one describing pressures in industry-sponsored clinical research and the other listing sample guidelines for practice (DHHS OIG, 2000c,d).

Shutdowns of Clinical Research at Academic and VA Medical Centers

In May 1999, OPRR halted human research studies at Duke University Medical Center, sending shock waves throughout the research community. Within a year, FDA and OPRR proceeded to halt all or some clinical research projects at seven other research centers.[5] These events focused the attention of research administrators on IRB operations and human subject protections with an intensity not seen in two decades. In November and December 2000, the newly established DHHS Office for Human Research Protections (OHRP)[6] issued "compliance determination" letters that found that studies in the intramural program at NIH were out of compliance with federal regulations. OPRR/OHRP has restricted or suspended multiple project assurances and required corrective actions at nearly a dozen academic institutions, and FDA has suspended clinical research at others.[7] OPRR/OHRP sanctions were imposed when numerous deficiencies and concerns regarding systemic protections for human subjects were found. Deficiencies occurred in such areas as IRB membership, education of IRB members and investigators, institutional commitment, initial and continuing review of protocols by IRBs, review of protocols involving vulnerable persons, and procedures for obtaining voluntary, informed consent. Also in 1999 it was discovered that researchers with the U.S. Department of Veterans Affairs (VA) in West Los Angeles were performing risky research without obtaining partici-

---

[5] OHRP maintains a list of "compliance determination" letters, indexed by month, on its website at http://ohrp.osophs.dhhs.gov/detrm_letrs/lindex.htm; FDA lists clinical researchers who have been sanctioned at http://www.fda.gov/ora/compliance_ref/bimo /dis_res_assur.htm; and the Office of Research Integrity lists debarred investigators at http://www.fda. gov/ora/compliance_ref/debar/default.htm.

[6] In June 1999, the Secretary of HHS created a new office, the Office for Human Research Protection (OHRP), to replace the Office for Protection from Research Risks (OPRR), which had been responsible for oversight of research involving human participants at institutions receiving federal funds and implementing the 18-agency federal Common Rule. The location of OPRR had been debated for years. Three background papers prepared for NBAC pointed to difficulties in having the office responsible for ethical conduct housed under the director for extramural research at National Institutes of Health (NIH), effectively subordinate to the funding office for extramural research, and poorly positioned to exert influence over the NIH intramural research program (Fletcher, forthcoming; Gunsalus, forthcoming; McCarthy, forthcoming). The NBAC papers all cited a need to elevate the administrative hub for protecting human research participants up and out of NIH, but differed in whether the location should be within DHHS or in an independent executive agency. A committee convened by then NIH Director Harold Varmus recommended in June 1999 that OPRR be moved to the level of the HHS Secretary and, among other things, that the Secretary create an external advisory committee for the office and that resources be increased for monitoring and enforcement (Office for Protection from Research Risks Review Panel, 1999). Less than six months after its creation, OHRP began a streamlined IRB registration and assurance process.

[7] Multiple project assurances are agreements between institutions and the federal government that pledge compliance with human subject regulations under 45 CFR 46. Suspension of these assurances effectively ceases research requiring IRB review. FDA actions include "clinical holds" on all or part of an institution's research under FDA human subject regulations (21 CFR 50, 21 CFR 56, and 21 CFR 312.120).

in West Los Angeles were performing risky research without obtaining participants' consent, leading to congressional hearings and a subsequent change in
VA policies (see below) (U.S. House of Representatives, Committee on Veterans Affairs, 1999).

The Death of Jesse Gelsinger

Attention was already focused on the protection of human research participants when 18-year-old Jesse Gelsinger died in a phase I gene transfer study at
the University of Pennsylvania in September 1999. He was a relatively healthy
(i.e., medically stable) young adult with a genetic condition—ornithine transcar-
bamylase deficiency—who had suffered intermittent health crises because of his
condition throughout his life but who was doing relatively well on medications
when he entered the gene transfer trial (Gelsinger, 2000; Lehrman, 2000a,b).
The details of the case are complex and to some extent contested. Although Gelsinger was aware that he was in a gene transfer study, the FDA found that the
consent form had been altered from that which had been approved and that data
relevant to safety had not been reported. Questions were raised about whether
some patients in the trial, including Gelsinger, fit the revised inclusion criteria
and whether the IRB and relevant federal agencies were notified of adverse
events that had occurred in studies with animals and in previous patients (Weiss
and Nelson, 1999).

The Gelsinger case was heavily reported in the national media and drew the
attention of clinical investigators and research administrators throughout the world.
It also became the focus of a Senate hearing and commanded direct attention from
the Secretary of HHS, who subsequently requested the Institute of Medicine (IOM)
study presented in this report (see discussion below) (Shalala, 2000; U.S. Senate,
Subcommittee on Public Health, Committee on Health, Education, Labor, and Pensions). Problems with the system of protections for those participating in research
were already apparent in 1999, but the Gelsinger death brought a sharp escalation in
attention because it resulted from the experimental intervention and failures in the
system of protections more than his underlying condition.

A CALL FOR ACCOUNTABILITY

The events of the 1990s that led to this report continuously highlighted the
need for reform of the system of protections for humans involved in research.
The rapid growth in the size of the research enterprise, the constant innovations
in experimental tools and approaches, and growing demands on the review process from the public and research sponsors alike led PRIM&R and others to ask
whether improvements could be gained by the establishment of standards for
systems for the protection of humans, accompanied by a method for the measurement of compliance. Others argue that current ethical principles codified in

the federal regulations and relevant international guidelines are sufficient. These observers argue that what is needed are more resources devoted to IRBs and regulatory agencies to ensure that protections are in place (Amdur, 2000; Snyderman and Holmes, 2000; Sugarman, 2000).

In 1999 and 2000, several groups moved forward with plans to develop standards for accreditation of IRBs and human research protection programs. These initiatives have come forward largely from two groups: one spawned from the PRIM&R effort and the other developed through a contract between NCQA and the VA. The origins of both are discussed in Chapter 2.

STATEMENT OF TASK

In October 2000, the Secretary of HHS asked the IOM to conduct a two-phase study to address three interrelated topics involved in the protection of human research subjects. The three topics are (1) accreditation standards for HRPPPs[8], (2) the overall structure and functioning of activities for the protection of human research subjects, including but not restricted to IRBs, and (3) criteria for evaluation of the performance of activities for the protection of human research subjects.

The IOM response is being conducted in two phases. Phase 1, the subject of this report, focuses on accreditation standards for HRPPPs. The specific tasks for phase 1 are to

1. review and consider proposed HRPPP performance standards;
2. recommend standards for accreditation of HRPPPs, considering measures of structure, process, and performance, as well as resource sufficiency; and
3. recommend steps that the organizations and institutions conducting research and the federal government should take to collect and analyze data to monitor and evaluate how well the system for protecting human subjects is operating.

Phase 2 will continue the 24-month study of the structure, function, and performance of activities for the protection of human research subjects.[9] The results of this future work will be presented as a separate report.

DEFINITIONS

In this section on definitions, the committee wishes to clarify its choice of terms to avoid confusion within this report and also to signal its awareness of the

---

[8] In the course of committee deliberations, the term "human research participant protection program" was substituted for "human research review program" as the former term better reflected the system of oversight that the committee hopes will result from its recommendations.

[9] For more information see http://www.iom.edu/hrrp.

semantic difficulties, which are related to substantive and theoretical differences. Three questions regarding terminology are addressed below: (1) what should individuals who volunteer to be part of a research study be called? (2) what elements and research contexts should be included in an HRPPP? and (3) what is accreditation?

Subject or Participant?

The committee received disparate, sometimes directly contradictory advice about what to call those individuals who participate in research but who are not investigators. Those studied in human research have been called "subjects," "participants," "patients," "respondents," "partners," "interviewees," "probands," "volunteers," and other terms. More recently, additional consideration has been given to the status of individuals who are identified by virtue of their relationship to the person who is the subject of the research, either because of biological or familial ties or because of membership in the same social, ethnic, or racial group. However, some of the terms apply only in a particular research context.

Federal regulations and international guidelines refer to "human subjects" of research. The reason for this language is to distinguish the person being studied from the investigator, to make clear who is the object of study, and to signal a power asymmetry. The framework underlying the regulations is to "protect" the rights and interests of subjects, with the underlying premise being that those being studied are vulnerable when their interests conflict with those of science or investigators. The regulations are intended to make clear that when such conflicts arise, the human rights of subjects trump the scientific interests of investigators and their institutions.

As discussed earlier, the initial framework for HRPPPs grew out of reaction against studies that put humans at risk for the benefit of science, particularly against their will or without their informed consent. It was natural to classify them as "human subjects," to emphasize the power and information asymmetries, but without intending to imply a passive or demeaning role. This concept was further extended by focusing on "vulnerable" populations especially prone to coercion or at higher risk, such as children, prisoners, pregnant women, and those with diminished mental capacities. The "human subject" framework was fully intended to pit individual rights against collective interests, and therein lay its value.

This framework of protection conflicts, however, with an alternative framework that sees research as a good in itself. Advocates (including prospective "human subjects") have come to regard access to research as a right. AIDS activists argued for "drugs into bodies" and fundamentally reframed the debate about the role of individuals in research participation (Epstein, 1996). The same shift has spilled over into debates about women in health research, breast cancer research, and research on ethnic groups, minorities, and underserved populations (Batt, 1994; IOM, 1994, 1999; Love, 1995; Merkatz and Summers, 1997).

Involvement in research is a topic of special sensitivity to at least some members of minority populations; and what to call those who volunteer for research is a matter of serious debate, but no consensus has been reached. At the committee's public forum, one African-American speaker strongly urged the committee to abandon the term "human subject" because it was demeaning, locked into place a policy framework that emphasizes powerlessness and passivity, and cast the discussion in the penumbra of the Tuskegee Study (Ashe, 2001). Advocates concerned about American Indians, breast cancer, and mental illness have reiterated this recommendation to the committee. Yet, it was an African-American legal scholar who argued for use of the word "subject" because it rightly emphasizes real-world vulnerabilities and comports with established regulatory language.

Debates about words reflect not just differences in referents but also differences in rhetorical purposes. The term "subject" highlights the reality of information and power imbalances, whereas the term "participants" or "partners" reflects a moral aspiration. One expresses subjects' need to be protected, but the other expresses the regard for participants' direct contribution and involvement in an ideal research system.

Underlying practical differences exist beyond these political and moral differences. A human subject in one study may be a seriously ill patient deciding among experimental treatments under the guidance of a health care professional. Yet the same regulations that cover the seriously ill patient cover a student of journalism interviewing prominent business figures, in which the "subject" may be considerably more powerful than the investigator, as well as those who respond to a survey (if it contains personal identifiers) and have only glancing contact with any investigator. Even within the confines of clinical trials for drugs, a person participating in the trial may truly be the healthy "subject" in whom a prospective drug is being tested for dose and toxicity, may be someone choosing among small twigs of an elaborate and extensive decision tree, or may be a desperately ill patient choosing among options that are all risky and experimental. Thus, no one word can fit snugly into all these situations.

NBAC devotes a section of its forthcoming oversight report to its choice of a term. In the end it has chosen to use the neutral word "participant" because it avoids some sensitivities and is unlikely to be confused with investigators in context. This choice has a cost in that it diverges from formal regulatory language and loses the immediate sense of vulnerability that the regulatory language was intended to signal. Most members of the present IOM committee nonetheless concur with NBAC's choice, "participant," primarily because many of the committee's recommendations reinforce the aspiration to involve participants more directly in research and its oversight. The committee will therefore refer to "participants" except in contexts in which a more precise term is preferred.

What Is a Human Research Participant Protection Program?

The current framework for HRPPPs grew out of research conducted by a single investigator at a single institution that could assign protocol review to a single IRB. With the expansion of the scope and scale of research and particularly the expansion of privately funded research, a growing fraction of research falls outside this research institution framework. If the research design comes from a central sponsor—whether it is an agency gathering statistical data on the national population, an NIH institute, or a private firm testing a drug or a device—the participants in a trial may be drawn from dozens or even hundreds of places. In addition, the study may involve many research institutions and go outside traditional research sites into clinics and community hospitals or even (as in the case of surveys) into the general population. The power of each individual institution and its associated IRBs is limited to that institution. Under the current system, each IRB makes a separate and distinct determination that results in approval, disapproval, or modification of a research study. Collectively, the IRB rulings for the same protocol may result in disparate or even contradictory findings.

The committee's first task was to make recommendations about accreditation standards for "human research participant protection programs," a term by implication (tautologically) defined to be the unit of accreditation. As discussed in Chapter 3, the proposed NCQA and PRIM&R standards essentially assume the unit of accreditation to be

- VA facilities to be accredited by NCQA; or
- research institutions that conduct biomedical research and that have one or more IRBs.

This committee uses the term to embrace a set of functions and institutions somewhat wider than those contemplated in the draft standards to include boards that monitor the safety of clinical trials or that report serious and unexpected adverse events that arise from research and also to include research organizations not configured as academic research institutions (Figure 1-1). The key components of HRPPPs are

- the organizational units responsible for designing, overseeing, and conducting research (which, for some research, includes research sponsors);
- the IRB reviewing that research;
- the investigators carrying out the research;
- monitoring bodies (including data safety and monitoring boards; ombudsman programs; data collection centers; and reporting mechanisms for adverse events, complaints, and concerns); and
- the participants involved in the research.

The term HRPPP and the various contexts in which it applies are further discussed below in an effort to clarify the scope of the committee's findings and recommendations.

The Centrality of Informed Consent

The first sentence of the Nuremberg Code is "The voluntary consent of the human subject is absolutely essential" (Nuremberg Code, 1949). To achieve this goal, the legal doctrine of informed consent was imported into research and medical care. The 1962 Kefauver-Harris Amendments made informed consent part of U.S. law by mandating that experimental drugs be used only if physicians obtained informed consent.[10] Informed consent relies on the triad of (1) a voluntary (uncoerced) choice (2) made by a person (or a formally designated surrogate) competent to do so and (3) informed by understanding of risks and potential benefits (Faden and Beauchamp, 1986). Informed consent is the centerpiece of the Common Rule and the focus of one of FDA's two main human subject protection regulations (21 CFR 50). IRBs spend more time and effort examining informed-consent documents than any other function (Bell et al., 1998), and the *process* of informed consent, to ensure that the three criteria above are met, is even more important than ensuring that informed-consent forms are clearly worded, signed, and archived. Informed consent is the bedrock for the ethical conduct of research.

Informed consent is therefore also the heart of HRPPPs. It is directly pertinent to accreditation standards and their use in the accreditation process because many of the most detailed aspects of federal regulations—and, consequently, of both NCQA and PRIM&R standards—deal with the documentation of informed consent. This is an area in which the standards may be most onerous and in which a shift to the use of performance measures—ways of getting and documenting genuine informed consent that do not rely as heavily on formal written, signed documents, as current practice does—would be most welcome. The current formal, "contractual" practice is one of the most alien to investigators and study participants in many foreign countries (Marshall, forthcoming), and *documentation* is one of the most nettlesome issues that breeds conflict between investigators and IRBs despite nearly universal acceptance of the underlying ethical principle.

The empirical literature about the informed-consent process, cultural variations in how to interpret the ethical conduct of research, and diverse methods for obtaining and documenting informed consent will be reviewed in the committee's subsequent report. Even before that report appears, however, the committee notes that retrieval and documentation of informed consent are essential and are required by federal regulations, but accreditation bodies should strive to permit and even encourage experimentation with alternative methods to ensure informed consent within the parameters of current regulations. The waiver authority already present in the regulations for research involving minimal risk to participants (45 CFR 46.117(c)) could be used to accumulate experience, with an eye to developing less

---

[10] Federal Food, Drug, and Cosmetic Act of 1938. P.L. No. 75-717, 52, Stat. 1040, as amended 21 U.S.C. 31 et seq.

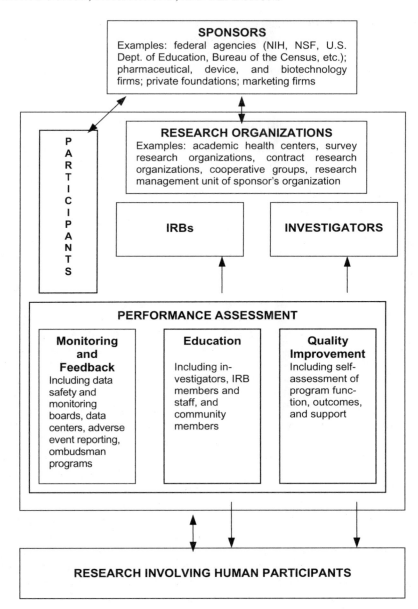

FIGURE 1-1 Human research participant protection programs. The components in the large box are all parts of an HRPPP. Arrows represent information flow pathways, not organizational responsibilities. All units within an HRPPP should have formalized communication procedures.

intrusive but equally valid methods for obtaining informed consent for research involving more than minimal risk. Such methods could, in turn, produce measures of informed consent that are more effective and less bureaucratic and that might eventually enable a shift in accreditation standards from documentation to assessment of genuine informed consent.

The Rise of Clinical Trials and Privately Funded Research

Clinical trials constitute only a subset of research, but they are an important subset. Clinical trials comprise a sizeable fraction of the studies that entail medical risks to participants and are a large and growing fraction of medical research. Also, on the basis of the growth of organizations dedicated to managing clinical trials and other evidence, it appears that the number of privately financed clinical trials has grown dramatically over the past decade (Rettig, 2000). Those trials conducted at a research institution with an HRPPP can be accommodated by attending explicitly to the roles and responsibilities of research sponsors. Many trials, however, are "multicenter trials" involving participants drawn from academic medical centers, private physicians' practices, community hospitals, clinics, and other institutions. Some of these may, in fact, lack an IRB.

In some cases, organizations that manage multicenter trials have developed, and these present a particular challenge to determination of the appropriate HRPPP unit. In cancer research, for example, several "oncology cooperative groups" have existed for decades to organize such trials, so that today 1,400 institutions participate. Community hospitals are also engaged in research through the Community Clinical Oncology Program, which includes 52 centers in 30 states (NCI, 1997): The National Cancer Institute is forming a central IRB and is revamping its support structure for clinical trials. This is driven in large part by the need to increase the scope and scale of clinical trials (NCI, 2001).

For multicenter trials, research sponsors are often very large organizations for which clinical trials are only a small fraction of their work (e.g., pharmaceutical firms or NIH institutes), and so the sponsor may not be the appropriate unit for HRPPP accreditation. When large organizations sponsor and conduct trials, however, they have organizational units that are responsible for trial oversight and that could apply for accreditation. In large multicenter trials, individual research institutions are at too low a level for meaningful accreditation because many such institutions are involved in the trial and none has meaningful control over the study design and overall safety. The appropriate locus of accreditation for multicenter clinical trials might prove to be different from that for research in general and might be focused on the organizations that have developed to manage the research, such as contract research organizations for privately funded trials or cooperative groups for both private and publicly funded trials. Accreditation bodies might devise a special set or subset of standards for such organizations.

Another option for multicenter trials is to focus on the IRB review step specifically. A research sponsor may pay for review by an IRB, constituted in compliance with FDA regulations for research involving human subjects but not affiliated with any particular research institution and not in control of the investigators, who are accountable instead to the research sponsor. Such organizations are discussed in further detail below.

Nonbiomedical Research

The committee heard about the potential problems of applying an oversight system designed to ensure the ethical conduct of clinical trials in medical research to other research methods. The United States requires review of federally funded research in disciplines outside medicine, but many other countries review only medical research. Although the principles of informed consent and the importance of oversight apply to all research, the principles will be applied in different ways when the risks are social rather than medical and when the goals of research may not be prevention, detection, or treatment of disease. Therefore, the risks and benefits of such projects will be analyzed differently from those of clinical trials, and such projects will require different kinds of expertise and sensitivities to different categories of research participants.

Research in anthropology, sociology, journalism, law, and economics, for example, requires distinct methods. Further, distinct methods and issues apply to the gathering and analysis of data for national statistical databases. Student projects at a college or graduate school or even a high school education research initiative do not map neatly to IRB review mechanisms at an academic medical center. Interviews, surveys, oral histories, and other methods common to the social sciences must be reviewed in light of expertise in relevant fields.

In response to the committee's call for public comments, the committee did not hear pleas to exempt nonmedical research from oversight, but several groups expressed concern that the draft accreditation standards (in this case, the PRIM&R standards) would require elaboration of formal policies and documentation that would be irrelevant for IRBs primarily reviewing social science, behavioral research, anthropology, sociology, oral history, epidemiology, and population studies (Levine, 2001; Overbey, 2001; Shopes, 2001). The committee did hear suggestions to reduce paperwork, to develop criteria sensitive to social and behavioral research, and to expand the categories of research exempt from review when the risks of nonmedical research are inherently low and informed consent can be "presumed" (e.g., by returning a survey form or answering questions in an interview) (Erickson, 2001; Rubin, 2001; Rudder, 2001).

Many of the policy options are relevant to the committee's subsequent report on the overall system of research oversight, but nonmedical research does raise some questions relevant to accreditation specifically. The American Association of University Professors has prepared a white paper on this topic

(AAUP, forthcoming), and the Committee on National Statistics, collaborating with the Board on Behavioral, Cognitive, and Sensory Sciences (National Research Council), is commencing a study of research oversight for the social and behavioral sciences that should inform the present IOM committee's subsequent report. The committee believes that in the meantime it will be important that emerging accreditation standards and the accreditation bodies that use them take this diversity of research into account and clearly indicate those mainly or solely applicable to clinical research (see further discussion in Chapter 2 and Recommendation 5).

Independent IRBs

The mandates and functions of independent IRBs are similar in scope to those of IRBs housed within an institution. Both types of review bodies and their administrative staffs function within a prescribed set of FDA regulations and according to guidance documents requiring initial review and protocol approval. Thereafter, ongoing review activities include monitoring of adverse events, oversight of recruitment activities, and review and approval of protocol amendments. The trend over the past decade has been for industry sponsors to conduct more multicenter studies outside of the institutional framework, thereby shifting the jurisdictional locus from the IRBs of individual institutions to independent (central) IRBs. Such boards review a growing fraction of research both in the United States and abroad. Thus, accreditation bodies need to develop standards or a subset of standards that embrace the independent IRB model.

Independent IRBs can stop a trial, but they do not employ investigators or have authority over them in the same way that the faculty at an academic health center does. The sections of the NCQA and PRIM&R draft standards on "research institutions" and "investigators" therefore do not apply directly to independent IRBs (Isidor, 2001). The operations of IRBs could, however, be accredited, and given their growing importance, independent IRBs should be included in any credible accreditation system. An independent IRB or group of IRBs administered by a single organization might be accredited, perhaps by using the subset of standards applicable to IRBs only, with oversight of investigators and the actual conduct of research performed through mechanisms other than accreditation (e.g., by FDA or OHRP review of sponsors and investigators). Accreditation of independent IRBs could be made contingent, for example, on ensuring that the sponsors from whom they accept work meet specific criteria. Sponsors should disclose whether a protocol has previously been disapproved by any IRB.

Most research reviewed by independent IRBs consists of clinical trials for drugs, devices, and biologics. Guidelines for the ethical conduct of such clinical trials already exist, however. These are the International Conference on Harmonisation Guidelines for Good Clinical Practice (ICH-GCP) which apply to any research conducted under an investigational new drug application (IND) subject to FDA approval. If sponsors are operating under an IND or otherwise agree to abide by ICH-GCP guidelines, particularly if those guidelines were strengthened to ensure a stronger voice for research participants, independent IRBs could be accredited for their capacity to do a thorough review, leaving oversight of research sponsors and investigators to FDA under existing regulations. Independent IRBs would be accredited only if they made their review contingent on the sponsors' agreement to ensure the ethical conduct of research under the sponsors' direct control, including the use of investigators who agree to abide by accepted standards.

Sponsors

To accredit HRPPPs as a system representing the complement of necessary activities that ensure the protection of human research participants, the responsibilities of research sponsors must also be included within the accreditation structure. Although existing FDA regulations, for example, assign the ultimate accountability for ensuring the management of ethical research to the sponsor, this does not alleviate the need for organizations seeking to run an HRPPP from incorporating this responsibility into their programs. In instances of clinical research involving drugs, devices, and other products under the purview of FDA regulations, the FDA would continue to be the locus of enforcement. Another option would be to consider organizational units within sponsoring organizations as the unit for accreditation, but this would be an entirely new strategy and would entail the use of accreditation strategies drastically different from those used in the accreditation models that the committee considered.

The Role of the Research Participant

Those in the best position to judge the interests of individuals participating in research are the participants themselves or informed representatives of participant perspectives. This is both a moral principle and a practical fact. The central tenet of the Nuremberg Code and the first principle of *The Belmont Report* center on individual autonomy, honoring Immanuel Kant's categorical imperative to "Act so that you treat humanity, whether your own person or another, always as an end and never as a means only" (Kant, 1999, p. 566). Those participating in research are also in the best position to appreciate their wants and needs as a practical matter, and the principle of autonomy suggests that their wishes should be respected (Faden and Beauchamp, 1986). Although participants are often not in a position to judge the scientific value of a protocol, participant perspectives can improve the study design, review of protocols, and oversight of ongoing research. They may identify procedures that add only marginal technical value but that cause serious inconvenience or increase the risk to participants. Study designs that accommodate participant needs can improve recruitment and retention of participants and thereby strengthen the study. The presence of representatives of study participants on study design and oversight panels also adds credibility to the review and monitoring processes among participants.[11]

Those developing accreditation standards would do well to directly involve focus groups, consent monitors, and participant representatives (e.g., those who themselves have been involved in past studies and who represent a genuine constituency) in specifying the desired outcomes to be incorporated into accreditation standards. In his book on accreditation, Michael Hamm cited the example of groups representing people with disabling conditions who were able to list desirable attributes of buildings that would permit access (Hamm, 1997). Participant involvement includes participation with the study design and representation on IRBs, monitoring bodies, and oversight and advisory bodies for research institutions.

Research Monitoring

Research monitoring was foremost among the problems identified by DHHS OIG (DHHS OIG, 1998a,b,c,d,e, 2000b,c,d). The main function of IRBs has been and will remain the review of protocols for proposed research to ensure that the research design is sound, that participants give their informed consent, and that selection of subjects is fair. IRBs are already busy with their current responsibilities, and research monitoring is an additional duty. IRBs therefore may not be the unit best able to carry out the monitoring of research. The committee believes that research monitoring—including adverse event reporting, data safety and monitoring boards, ombudsman programs, reporting mechanisms for concerns or complaints, and consent monitoring programs—should be defined as part of an HRPPP but not laid solely at the feet of the IRB component of an HRPPP.

The significant role of research monitoring is evident through the many elements of the ICH-GCP guidelines that relate to reporting of adverse events and other aspects of research monitoring. Research under an FDA IND must comply with strict reporting requirements for adverse events, and the federal code requires reporting of "unanticipated problems posing risks to subjects.".[12] Research monitoring is incorporated into NCQA standards but is not a central theme of the proposed PRIM&R standards, in which it is mentioned in only one documentation standard. The committee believes that adverse event reporting and research moni-

---

[11] Involvement of the National Breast Cancer Coalition was instrumental, for example, in clinical trials of the drug herceptin, when early clinical trials were having difficulty recruiting participants. The National Breast Cancer Coalition became involved, however, only when it could directly participate in trial design and oversight (Bazell, 1998).

[12] 45 CFR 46.103 (b)(5).

toring should be central elements of the system as a whole and, hence, also of any accreditation process intended to improve that system.

Accreditation Versus Certification

The committee uses the term "accreditation" to refer to a process described in Chapters 2 and 3. That process is centered on an organization rather than individuals. The committee uses the term "certification" to refer to an individual. The National Association of IRB Managers, for example, has offered a certification examination since 1995, and the Applied Research Ethics National Association recently has launched a certification program for individuals who staff or chair IRBs (National Association of IRB Managers, 2001; PRIM&R, 2001a).

Certification is offered only to those with demonstrated experience and entails passing a test of knowledge about protection of human research participants. Certification has been discussed for investigators who conduct research involving human participants. For example, the government of the United Kingdom licenses those doing animal research and research on in vitro fertilization and embryo research. In the United States, however, no structure to carry out national certification of U.S. investigators exists. NIH and several universities (e.g., Case Western Reserve University and the University of Rochester), for example, have recently adopted requirements that investigators take a World Wide Web-based interactive test that demonstrates knowledge of human research protections before they can seek IRB approval of a protocol (Case Western Reserve University, 2001; Chadwick and Liders, 2000; Office of Human Subjects Research, National Institutes of Health, 2001). A national certification requirement for investigators, however, would be a major step entailing the development of a substantial infrastructure. For this reason, the committee does not consider the issue of certification in this report.

2

Models of Accreditation

The committee was presented with the task of making recommendations about accreditation standards and does so in more detail in the next chapter. With the basic terminology for the committee's view of a human research participant protection program (HRPPP) defined in Chapter 1, this chapter lays the groundwork for the elements of an accreditation process. It starts by considering the various models available for accreditation systems and asks, "What is the role of accreditation in a human research protection system?" The present committee will spend another year thinking about the design and implementation of an improved system of human research protection, so it has not had the opportunity to consider the value of accreditation compared with other strategies to ensure the ethical conduct of research. However, even if one begins with the current system rather than a reconstructed one, accreditation should not be evaluated in a vacuum—it is still necessary to have a theory of accreditation and a process for carrying it out. Specifically, the value that accreditation adds to the system that already exists must be considered.

MODELS OF ACCREDITATION

Accreditation efforts in the United States have historically followed one of two models, although a third model can also be observed. The first of these is accreditation as a supplement to government regulation. Under this model, entities that are otherwise already regulated by the government seek accreditation as a mark of excellence, as it is above and beyond government regulation. Accreditation, however, has become a mark of excellence achieved by only a fraction of regulated entities.

The National Committee for Quality Assurance (NCQA) program for the accreditation of managed care organizations illustrates this model (NCQA, 2001a). Managed care organizations are regulated by state insurance departments, state health departments, or the U.S. Department of Health and Human Services (DHHS) (if they are Medicare or Medicaid managed care organizations). They also seek accreditation, however, to demonstrate their commitment to excellence, as many employers and other purchasers of managed care organization services look to accreditation as an indicator of performance above the required minimum.

In a second model, accreditation substitutes private regulation for public regulation. One version of this is seen in accreditation of institutions of higher education, for which formal government regulation is (for various reasons not explored here) largely absent. Accreditation serves effectively as the only oversight system.

Another variant of nongovernmental voluntary accreditation is seen under Medicare's "deemed-status" program, in which the Joint Commission on Accreditation of Healthcare Organizations (JCAHO) hospital accreditation program serves as an alternative to state certification, which uses Medicare's own federal regulatory standards as a basis for hospital participation in Medicare (Jost, 1994). JCAHO's accreditation standards are quite different from Medicare's own standards, but JCAHO accreditation is accepted in the place of Medicare certification. That is, a hospital or health care facility is deemed to meet federal standards by dint of being accredited by JCAHO and is thereby authorized to participate in (and be paid through) Medicare.

There are significant benefits to the use of accreditation as an alternative to regulation and to the deemed-status model in particular. Accreditation reduces the cost of oversight to government, as it is effectively paid for by user fees rather than taxes. Accreditation programs, especially nongovernmental programs, tend to be much more flexible and responsive to change than regulatory programs because they are not bound by the rigidities of administrative rule-making procedures and are more responsive to regulated constituencies. Accreditation, however, also has its costs. It is not directly accountable to the public, and there is a constant concern that the "fox is guarding the henhouse" (DHHS OIG, 1999a,b). Even JCAHO is not given unfettered authority to regulate hospitals for Medicare. The Health Care Financing Administration (HCFA), which administers Medicare, retains authority to directly assess (or "look behind") the accreditation of hospitals. HCFA conducts its own surveys for cause, surveying a small fraction of validation surveys each year, and reviews JCAHO's "deeming" authority at least once every 6 years (Lewin Group, 1998). Furthermore, if accreditation is to be more than a pro forma exercise, it can be resource-intensive. This can be corroborated by any health care facility or educational administrator who has recently undergone accreditation.

In a third, less common, model, the accreditation program does not create its own standards but, rather, ensures compliance with standards on the basis of interpretation of regulatory standards determined by the government or another entity. The program might also offer guidance about regulatory compliance. This is the accreditation model used by the Association for Assessment and Accreditation of Laboratory Animal Care (AAALAC),[1] which does not create its own standards but which is a private voluntary accreditation system that operates in compliance with regulations from the U.S. Department of Agriculture, funding agencies, and the Animal Welfare Act, a federal statute. AAALAC standards are supplemented by the *Guide for the Care and Use of Laboratory Animals,* produced by the National Research Council (NRC, 1996). This volume lays out best practices and benchmarks based on science and knowledge developed from past accreditation efforts.

AAALAC dates back to 1965. Until recently, the National Institutes of Health (NIH) office that had oversight over protection of humans involved in research also had responsibility for compliance with animal care regulations, so this model is familiar to both the federal officials and research centers. This is the model explicitly cited by the Association for the Accreditation of Human Research Protection Programs (AAHRPP) (see below). The analogy is not direct in one area, however, in that in research involving humans, participants can have a direct voice and those with direct experience as participants or those familiar with the concerns of human participants in research can be directly engaged in oversight of the research. The draft standards that the committee has seen to date do not fully take advantage of this possibility (see discussions in Chapters 1 and 3).

On the basis of the standards shared with the committee, it appears that the framework proposed by NCQA under its contract with the U.S. Department of Veterans Affairs (VA), at least initially, is to use accreditation as a tool to implement existing regulations better, adopting this aspect of the AAALAC model (in effect, using current regulations as standards and using accreditation to bring VA facilities into compliance with them). The committee believes that this is a good way in which to get an accreditation program under way. It might also serve to supplement a regulatory program that is overburdened. Its main value is to move those being accredited into compliance with existing regulations. This strategy will improve research oversight only if noncompliance is one of the system's major problems. The same model could, however, also be used to augment regulatory standards if some accreditation standards exceed the regulatory minimum. The NCQA linkage to quality improvement programs is a step along this path (see Chapter 3).

---

[1] For more information, see http://www.aaalac.org/.

ELEMENTS OF AN ACCREDITATION PROCESS

At the beginning of the 20th century, a private voluntary accreditation system lifted American medical education out of mediocrity. In the early 1900s, the quality and content of medical education were wildly variable. Harvard University, the University of Pennsylvania, and The Johns Hopkins University had instituted formal curricula and linked medicine to science, but "the ports of entry into medicine were wide open, and the unwelcome passed through in great numbers" (Starr, 1982, p. 116). The American Medical Association (AMA) appointed individuals from esteemed medical schools to the Council on Medical Education, and these individuals began to grade medical schools. A 1910 report by Abraham Flexner went a step further, arguing that the strategy for improving the system of medical education was by elevating schools to the Hopkins standard, and "the AMA Council effectively became a national accreditation agency for medical schools, as an increasing number of states adopted its judgments of unacceptable institutions" (Starr, 1982, p. 121).

Since then accreditation programs have been used to enhance quality in many different contexts. The improvement of care for laboratory animals involved in research has been widely attributed to the joint action of federal law, particularly the Animal Welfare Act of 1966, and the private accreditation system through AAALAC. Private accreditation has become pervasive in higher education and professional schools, hospitals and health care facilities, and managed care organizations. More recently, a long-standing and rigid regulatory framework for opioid treatment programs has begun to shift to a more flexible, clinically oriented accreditation process, even though it is still formally under federal regulation. An accreditation process is now proposed for HRPPPs.

The models described above have in common several elements that are expected to be part of emerging programs for accreditation of HRPPPs:

- a national organization that can mediate the accreditation process;
- an application process and set of threshold criteria by which organizations are eligible to apply for accreditation;
- a process of self-evaluation;
- an external evaluation process, including site visits by external accreditors;
- an appeals process for accreditation determinations;
- a repeat cycle of self-evaluation and external evaluation; and
- a set of standards by which HRPPPs can be measured.

The central focus of this report and the following chapter is accreditation standards, the benchmarks by which accreditation programs measure achievement. Standards are only part of a process, however. This chapter describes the accreditation process for which standards are a tool.

Accreditation Bodies

The committee believes that the ideal accreditation body is a national independent organization that is credible among the stakeholders to be accredited but that is independent of any particular interest group among them. Independence, credibility, and intimate familiarity with stakeholders' needs are desirable attributes of any accrediting body (Hamm, 1997), and particularly so for human participant protections. As described below, both NCQA and the emergent AAHRPP appear to meet these criteria.

PRIM&R and the Formation of AAHRPP

Public Responsibility in Medicine and Research (PRIM&R) is a Boston-based private nonprofit organization best known for its activities in educating institutional review board (IRB) members and staff.[2] It was founded in 1974, the same year in which the first bioethics commission, the National Commission for the Protection of Human Subjects of Biomedical and Behavioral Research (the National Commission), began its work. The framework for IRBs was not fully in place, but IRBs were already operating at NIH and in many academic health centers.

In 1999, PRIM&R formed a working group to develop accreditation standards. This grew out of discussions about the development of an accreditation process for HRPPPs (see Chapter 1), the organizational units responsible for carrying out the twin functions described by the National Bioethics Advisory Commission (NBAC) of ensuring informed consent and independently assessing risks and benefits. Under a subcontract executed for the purposes of the present committee's work, a preliminary draft of the PRIM&R standards was given to the Institute of Medicine (IOM) in December 2000 and became the focus of a January 2001 IOM public forum on the topic of accreditation standards. PRIM&R revised its draft standards after the public forum, and they appear in Appendix B. PRIM&R's proposed standards were a major input into the committee's deliberations and are discussed in greater detail in Chapter 3.

The concept of AAHRPP was originally conceived by PRIM&R and was intended to provide the organizational locus for carrying out an accreditation process by using the PRIM&R standards. AAHRPP is designed to bring together diverse stakeholder organizations with the intent of implementing a voluntary accreditation process. AAHRPP was originally incorporated in Massachusetts in March 2000, but it is expected to be incorporated in Maryland in spring 2001 as a private nonprofit corporation to "provide a process of voluntary peer review and education among organizations concerned with research involving human subjects, in order to promote preservation of rights and welfare of subjects in research and

---

[2] For more information, see http://www.primr.org.

compliance with relevant regulatory and ethical standards" (PRIM&R, 2001b). As this report went to press, AAHRPP was supported by a consortium of interested groups, including PRIM&R, the Association of American Medical Colleges (AAMC), the Association of American Universities, the Federation of American Societies for Experimental Biology, the National Health Council, the National Association of State Universities and Land Grant Colleges, and the Consortium of Social Science Organizations (Accrediting Body for Human Subjects Research Nears Reality, 2001).

The VA and NCQA Accreditation Process

In March 1999, clinical research at the West Los Angeles VA Medical Facility was suspended because of noncompliance with the Common Rule (see Chapter 1). In the ensuing months four additional VA medical centers were affected by Food and Drug Administration (FDA) or Office for Protection from Research Risks (OPRR) sanctions. This shone a spotlight on Veterans Affairs, just as OPRR and FDA shutdowns had done at other academic health centers. In April 1999, the VA announced the formation of a national office, the Office of Research Compliance and Assurance. In June 1999, the General Accounting Office commenced a study of human subject protections at VA medical centers and made eight site visits (GAO, 2000). That report identified three specific weaknesses: "(1) VA headquarters has not provided medical center research staff with adequate guidance about human subject protections; (2) insufficient monitoring and oversight of local human subject protections; and (3) insufficient funds allocated for IRB operations and human subject protection oversight" (p. 5).

To address these deficiencies, the VA awarded a $5.8 million, 5-year contract to establish a national accreditation system for VA medical centers engaged in research (VA, 2000). The contract was awarded to NCQA, which then began to devise and carry out an accreditation and oversight process (NCQA, 2001b). NCQA has joined with Medical Care Management Corporation (MCMC) to design the program and to recruit, credential, and schedule surveyors. NCQA and MCMC together will provide a routine external evaluation of compliance with policies.

In addition, NCQA plans to convene two advisory groups and one decision-making group to help develop and implement standards and survey methods for the program. NCQA presented the rationale behind its approach at IOM's January 2001 public forum and later provided the committee with a set of its draft standards (see Chapter 3 and Appendix C).

Private consulting and management firms such as Deloitte & Touche and PricewaterhouseCoopers have been hiring staff with HRPPP expertise and may assist with preparations for accreditation efforts. Other organizations may yet step forward to offer accreditation for HRPPPs.

Eligibility Criteria and an Application Process

The accreditation body must specify who can be accredited, set fees to cover its costs, and establish an application process. The NCQA accreditation of VA facilities will be done, at least initially, by self-selection. Because the VA hospital system is relatively closed, the applicant pool is clear. The eligibility criteria for HRPPPs beyond VA, including the nascent AAHRPP, have not been specified in detail. It is clear that academic or independent research centers that have an operating IRB would be eligible. The stated intention is to also invite applications from private independent IRBs. It is not clear whether larger consortia of institutions that are organized as a collaborative unit would be eligible, such as cooperative clinical trials groups,[3] the Multi-Center Academic Clinical Research Organization,[4] independent contract research organizations, or site management organizations.

Self-Evaluation

Applying for accreditation requires considerable preparation. This typically involves the organization that is seeking accreditation to gather information relevant to the standards that will be used and to analyze how well prepared it is to address questions and concerns that may arise. This preparation can consume enormous efforts of a few staff members and draws on the resources of many parts of the organization. The mere process of self-study can reveal previously unknown weaknesses or sometimes strengths and can suggest administrative remedies. It can also draw the attention of senior administrators to the need for more resources, new programs, or management changes and can reveal the strengths and weaknesses of key personnel. Many organizations involved in accreditation processes regard the self-study as the most valuable element of the accreditation process precisely because it focuses the attention of senior administrators.

The process of self-evaluation of HRPPPs appears to be especially promising as a way to improve the system. Self-assessment combined with systematic, continual use of quality improvement programs could, for example, identify features common to many "excellent" HRPPPs, and those features could, over

---

[3] The Office for Human Research Protections maintains a list of cooperative protocol research programs that might be accredited, but for which a somewhat different process and set of standards would be required. (For more information see http://ohrp.osophs.dhhs.gov/humansubjects/assurance/cprp.htm).

[4] Multi-Center Academic Clinical Research Organization, or MACRO, brings together five major academic health centers—Baylor College of Medicine, Harvard Clinical Research Institute, the University of Pennsylvania School of Medicine, Vanderbilt University, and Washington University School of Medicine—under a collaborative agreement that includes an agreed upon system for protocol review by IRBs among the institutions (for more information, see http://www.mc.vanderbilt.edu/ctc/macro.html).

time, supplant the existing regulatory standards, with their focus on IRB structure and documentation procedures. A shift from documentation-based standards to performance-based standards could not take place quickly, but it may well become possible over time (see Recommendations 6 and 7).

External Evaluation

The accreditation programs of NCQA and AAHRPP both intend to visit every organization seeking accreditation, at least initially. The accreditors visiting sites would review the self-evaluation; view documentation; and carry out interviews of IRB staff and members, administrators, investigators, and (if the recommendations of this IOM committee are adopted) participants. The site visit is intended to give accreditors a hands-on feel for the organization and to raise questions when they can be answered directly and immediately. The accreditors would then prepare a formal written report and make their decision to accredit the applicant, give it a probationary status, or reject the application.

Launching the accreditation process is likely to encounter some capacity limits for external evaluation. The committee concurs that site visits will be necessary initially, which will limit the number of institutions that can be accredited. At the committee's December 18 open meeting, David Korn of AAMC, which is involved with helping to establish AAHRPP, estimated that AAHRPP might eventually be able to accredit as many as 650 to 700 HRPPPs, but it would take a number of years to reach this level. This is one reason that the committee believes that the accreditation process should be regarded as a pilot study rather than a fait accompli (see Recommendation 1 below).

PRIM&R does have a core set of trained IRB professionals to draw upon for the initial AAHRPP site visits. This pool is limited, however, and it would be unrealistic to expect a new accreditation organization to manage more than one or two site visits per week, on average, during its first year. The minimum of potential applicants can be estimated by the 165 institutions that registered their IRBs with the Office for Human Research Protections (OHRP) as of February 5, 2001.[5] It appears likely, therefore, that it would take 2 to 3 years to accredit just those institutions that registered their IRBs in the first 2 months in which they were able to do so. It would take even longer to accredit the 491 institutions surveyed in 1995 in the most recent and extensive survey of IRB operations (Bell et al., 1998).

---

[5] The registration process began in December 2000. Most institutions have more than one IRB, so the number of IRBs registered is much larger than the number of potential applicant institutions.

Appeals Process

Institutions that fail to get accredited or that are given probationary status will need a credible appeals process. This may be through the accreditation body itself or may require some involvement of FDA or OHRP.[6] The NCQA standards include a standard for an appeals process by the applicant institution; the PRIM&R standards do not.

Repeat Accreditation

Accreditation is not permanent. The models of accreditation reviewed by the Lewin Group in 1998 involved accreditation terms of 3 to 5 years. The NCQA program plans a 3-year accreditation cycle. The AAHRPP accreditation term has not yet been firmly specified, but it is expected to be 3 to 5 years. The process for reapplication might or might not differ from that for initial accreditation. It is likely that accredited organizations with few untoward events would face a more abbreviated process, but this is likely to be decided in light of experience.

APPLYING THE MODELS TO HUMAN RESEARCH OVERSIGHT

Recommendation 1: Pursue Accreditation Through Pilot Testing as One Approach.

Accreditation of HRPPPs should be pursued as *one* promising approach to improving the human participant protection system. The first step is implementation of pilot programs to test standards, establish accreditation processes, and build confidence in accreditation organizations. This effort should be evaluated for its impact on protecting the rights and interests of participants in 3 to 5 years.

Accreditation as a mark of excellence—of achievement well beyond regulatory compliance—might offer an HRPPP a competitive advantage over nonaccredited competitors in seeking support from sponsors or access to participants, researchers, or students. That is, NIH or other funding review committees might look more favorably on research proposals from accredited institutions than on those from nonaccredited ones, those recruiting participants might advertise accreditation as a hallmark of quality and safety, or private drug and device firms might preferentially site clinical trials that they sponsor at accredited research institutions (or have them reviewed by accredited IRBs).

---

[6] For example, mammography accreditation entails a two-layer appeals process, first to the private body, but if it is denied, then the private body's decision can be appealed directly to FDA (Lewin Group, 1998).

Accreditation might also serve as an important educational tool. The process of preparing for accreditation would force institutions to attend to their HRPPPs, and that attention would necessarily entail education about the importance of protection of human participants in research. Accreditation could raise the median performance (average middle performance) of HRPPPs. It might offer HRPPPs located within research institutions, both public and private, a potent argument when asking their administrative supervisors for additional resources. (This is a major role played by accreditation of academic units within a university and is used as a tool to effect changes in, for example, library services, curricula, and services.) Accreditation could not serve these ends, however, until it became widely accepted as a mark of excellence. Any accreditation program seeking to establish its value on the basis of these terms would first need to achieve broad recognition as a credible program. All previous accreditation programs faced a similar dilemma when they were initiated, and some have succeeded in attaining credibility, but others have not.[7]

Accreditation that would supplant regulation (the deemed-status model) could have several attractive features. Both OHRP and FDA have signaled that they might consider accreditation by a nongovernmental accreditation organization presumptive evidence of compliance with regulations. In the case of research institutions under OHRP oversight, accreditation could serve as a partial substitute for the assurance and compliance functions, reducing FDA and OHRP scrutiny of accredited organizations (allowing them to concentrate their scrutiny on nonaccredited organizations). FDA and OHRP would necessarily retain independent oversight authority (e.g., inspections "for cause") and independent investigation and enforcement capacity if violations are alleged or documented and would periodically need to "accredit the accreditors," as in other deemed-status accreditation models. However, before the usefulness of this approach can be assessed in the case of HRPPP accreditation, an accreditation program(s) will need to be much further along in its development.

The regulatory enforcement model is also worth considering, particularly as a starting point. It might be wise to start, as NCQA apparently proposes to do under its contract with the VA, with a focus on innovative or more effective means of evaluating regulatory compliance before moving on to a program that raises standards above the regulatory minimum. This approach could, however, have the effect of inundating HRPPPs with further paperwork if additional requirements are imposed on current ones. If the goal is to shift from a focus on such paper compliance to a focus on more meaningful performance measures,

---

[7] Some accreditation programs fail to take root and flourish. An AMA physician certification program was announced with great fanfare in late 1996, but AMA discontinued the program in April 2000 because it had not been widely adopted. JCAHO implemented an accreditation program for managed care in 1987 but stopped in 1990, until a new managed care accreditation program was put in place in 1995 (BNA, 1996, 2000; Dimmitt, 1995).

then a strategy that assumes that current oversight is the baseline will not accomplish it and any additional measures will add to the regulatory burden. Again, it is important to look carefully at what value accreditation adds to the regulatory program that already exists and whether this added value justifies the added costs (financial and personnel) of such a program.

Testimony that the committee heard from representatives of the FDA and OHRP left it uncertain about whether the draft accreditation standards are seen as supplementing a regulatory program that will continue largely as is or as providing an alternative means of oversight, with federal agencies "deeming" accredited HRPPPs to be in compliance and thus reducing federal inspections and audits of accredited institutions.

A voluntary national accreditation system, however, could decrease the burden currently experienced by regulators, allowing them to refocus their efforts where they are most needed, and it could also increase flexibility for entities attempting regulatory compliance. An independent accreditation organization(s) could more readily modify and improve its standards than federal agencies carrying out mandatory programs. Federal agencies attempting to modify their regulatory approach are less flexible because they must follow formal rule-making procedures to do so. It took a decade to reach agreement on the federal Common Rule, and at least three agencies that conduct research with human participants did not adopt the rule,[8] leaving all agencies loathe to reopen the process used to modify the regulations. The current need for multiagency concurrence is a tremendous barrier, and so short-term improvements are more likely to come from other approaches, such as nongovernmental accreditation, that do not require major regulatory overhaul.[9]

The most compelling argument in favor of an independent accreditation system, however, is that, if it is done right, it could move the focus of oversight from simple administrative documentation to focusing on processes and outcomes that more directly threaten the rights and interests of participants. The need to shift from paper compliance to measures that more meaningfully prevent unnecessary risks, promote sound scientific design, and ensure autonomous choice has been a consensus direction for improvement since regulations were first implemented. The call for better measures was articulated by the President's Commission for the Study of Ethical Problems in Medicine and Biomedical and

---

[8] OPRR noted three agencies that appeared to sponsor research with human participants but that were not signatories to the Common Rule: the National Endowment for the Humanities, the U.S. Department of Labor, and the Nuclear Regulatory Commission, as cited in a report forthcoming from NBAC (NBAC, forthcoming-b).

[9] The rigidity of the current regulatory framework, entailing the consensus of 18 agencies, is one major argument that NBAC offers to support its recommendation for new legislation to create a single federal agency with oversight authority for protection of human participants in research. This topic is beyond the scope of this committee's first report but will likely be taken up in its subsequent report.

Behavioral Research (the President's Commission) in reviewing regulations created in the wake of the National Commission and echoed in reports of the Advisory Committee on Human Radiation Experiments (ACHRE) in 1995 and the Office of the Inspector General (OIG) of DHHS in 1998 and 2000 (ACHRE, 1995; DHHS OIG, 1998a,b,c,d, 2000a,b,c; President's Commission, 1981, 1983).

Recommendation 2: Establish a Nongovernmental Accreditation Organization(s).

Organizations formulating accreditation standards and carrying out the accreditation process should be independent, nongovernmental organizations. These organizations should include within their programmatic leaderships the perspective of the relevant stakeholders in the applicant HRPPP community (i.e., institutions, investigators, sponsors, and participants).

As discussed above, one of the chief virtues of a nongovernmental accreditation system is that it can evolve over time without requiring new federal regulations at each step. The regulations are demonstrably unresponsive to dramatic changes in how research is conducted; a nongovernmental accreditation system may be more responsive by comparison and would comport with Circular A-119 of the Office of Management and Budget, which urges the use of nongovernmental "voluntary consensus standards" where possible (OMB, 1998).[10]

The committee envisions an accreditation process that will continually evolve to update standards over time and to incorporate the variety of organizational structures through which human research programs are reviewed and carried out. The operations of organizations seeking accreditation will also evolve. The parallel evolution of accreditation standards and HRPPP operations should be an iterative process, with the formulation of standards efficiently informed by knowledge acquired in the accreditation process. The formulation of standards, the conduct of accreditation site visits, and external evaluation must therefore be intimately linked and appropriately responsive to feedback.

Organizations formulating standards and conducting the accreditation process should

1. be national in scope;

2. be familiar with the operations of institutions that apply for accreditation; and

3. incorporate the perspectives of research participants within their programmatic leaderships.

---

[10] Circular A-119 was intended mainly for technical standards pertaining to products, but it also contemplates "related management systems practices" (see http://www.whitehouse.gov/omb/circulars/a119/a119.html).

An accreditation process should directly involve the kinds of institutions and research expertise being accredited, but an accreditation organization should not be beholden to any particular stakeholder or interest group. Accreditation bodies for HRPPPs will require input from academic health centers, organizations representing research sponsors, nongovernmental research organizations, private firms developing products and services tested in studies with humans, participants, IRB members and staff from both academic and nonacademic institutions, research administrators in both academic and nonacademic institutions, and individuals from a range of research fields appropriate to the intended range of applicant institutions.

SOME ISSUES THAT ACCREDITATION ALONE CANNOT ADDRESS

Some elements important to the protection of the rights and interests of those participating in research are not directly addressed in proposed programs for HRPPP accreditation. In most cases, an accreditation process could be used as an indirect means to improvement; however, further actions would be needed in parallel with the establishment of an accreditation process. The committee expects to come back to many of these topics in its second report and has discussed how to integrate some elements not currently emphasized into the accreditation process. The discussion below includes some suggestions to that effect.

Accreditation is not a short-term fix. It must be viewed as one element of a long-term strategy. The VA-NCQA accreditation program will operate in a relatively circumscribed system, but it will take several years to implement the system and several more to evaluate it. The national voluntary system being developed under AAHRPP may take even longer to establish. Before a program could be granted deemed status it would need to be given time to develop and mature. Turning over regulatory authority to an untested program would be very risky, reinforcing the need for pilot testing as a first step.

Identifying, Investigating, and Sanctioning Violations

Accreditation cannot totally replace federal regulation. Accreditation is rarely effective in dealing with bad actors—those who intentionally flout or ignore requirements. Monitoring, investigation, and enforcement are necessary to augment an accreditation system, and under the current regulatory framework these will remain functions of OHRP and the FDA.[11] The main cause of error in many prominent controversies in research ethics lies with investigators who diverge from an agreed-upon protocol. Review of protocols cannot fix the prob-

---

[11] One recommendation of NBAC is to consolidate these functions into a single agency, as noted above.

lem when investigators deviate from the protocols, although a more robust research monitoring capacity could reduce such deviations. Some of the most conspicuous cases in the past two decades—Martin Cline's 1980 gene transfer experiments in Israel and Italy (Thompson, 1994) and the death of Jesse Gelsinger in gene transfer experiments at the University of Pennsylvania in 1999, for example[12]—appear to be attributable to the conduct of principal investigators and their collaborators or to institutional decisions unrelated to the IRB, so it is not clear how accreditation of an HRPPP could prevent such cases.

An accreditation body should not be expected to be the original source responsible for uncovering violations or the main body responsible for investigating or sanctioning them. Accreditation could, over time, reduce the likelihood that violations would occur as a result of changes in norms and behaviors. Accreditation could, moreover, be withdrawn or made probationary on the basis of the disclosure of infractions at an accredited institution. Reports of infractions would surely increase scrutiny by an accreditation body. An accreditation organization could also be used as part of the strategy to bring an institution back into compliance with federal regulations after infractions were detected and investigated. Therefore, accreditation is relevant to the problem of bad actors, but

---

[12] In 1980, Martin Cline administered recombinant DNA with the hope of effecting gene transfer in two patients with thalassemia, one in Israel and one in Italy. His IRB had not approved his protocol and, indeed, rejected it just days after Cline conducted the experiments. The IRB had reviewed the protocol several times and had enlisted external expert reviewers who uniformly judged the experiment premature. Cline also deliberately misled a review panel in Israel and his collaborator in Italy, who identified the patient who was treated. The experiments had no known adverse health consequences for the patients, and after an NIH investigation, Cline had several grants terminated and was barred from seeking NIH funds for 4 years; he also resigned from his division chairmanship at the University of California at Los Angeles. IRB action in connection with this protocol was not at fault in the infractions. This case was reviewed in Larry Thompson's *Correcting the Code* (Thompson, 1994) and in a background paper for NBAC (Cook-Deegan, 1997).

IRB action was similarly a relatively minor concern in the 1999 death of Jesse Gelsinger. The lawsuit brought by his family focuses on the actions of the principal investigator and two research institutions: James Wilson, a private company (Genovo), and the Institute for Human Gene Therapy at the University of Pennsylvania. Arthur Caplan, a bioethicist who gave advice about the trial design, was initially also named in the suit, but he was not on the IRB. Actions named in the suit, which was settled out of court on terms that have not been publicly disclosed, focus mainly on deviations from the protocol approved by the IRB and not on IRB actions. The only mention of the IRB is that it approved the protocol (for more information, see http://www.sskrplaw.com/links/healthcare2.html). The broader definition of an HRPPP could reduce the likelihood of similar events, particularly if the committee's recommendations about incorporating research monitoring were adopted.

it is not the most direct solution to the problem and cannot replace investigation and enforcement activities.

Educating Investigators

In 1995 ACHRE completed a report that built on a thorough historical and ethical analysis. It concluded:

> It is not clear to the Advisory Committee that scientists whose research involves human subjects are any more familiar with *The Belmont Report* today than their colleagues were with the Nuremberg Code forty years ago. . . . No one in the scientific community should be able to say "I didn't know" or "nobody told me" about the substance and importance of research ethics (ACHRE, 1995, pp. 817–818).

Many, perhaps most, of the serious problems that arise in human research arise from the actions of investigators, so policies that deal directly with investigators are at least as important as improving the review of research protocols in an HRPPP. The policies that most directly affect investigators include the following: educating them about their roles and responsibilities in the ethical conduct of research, increasing the capacity to monitor ongoing research approved by an IRB, the investigation of infractions, and the enforcement of regulations. Among these, education seems to be the one most likely to have the desired results with the least level of intrusion and the greatest direct impact on overall norms.

In a background paper written for NBAC, Charles McCarthy, drawing on two decades of direct experience with federal oversight of protection of human participants in research, argued that the measure most important to improving the ethical conduct of research is education—of investigators, IRB members, IRB staff, and those working at research institutions (McCarthy, forthcoming). The devotion of resources to education led to fewer problems down the road. Incidents requiring investigation and the need for intervention increased when budgets for education decreased, and increased attention to education seemed to reduce the numbers of untoward incidents.

McCarthy's observation is corroborated by the observations of ACHRE (Mastroianni and Kahn, 1998). Henry Beecher, in a seminal 1966 *New England Journal of Medicine* article, argued against establishing an oversight bureaucracy for medical research, asserting that the key was instead to elevate norms of research ethics among investigators (Beecher, 1966). The present committee concurs with that position.

Although accreditation can reinforce education programs at accredited institutions, education on the ethical conduct of research and the ethical responsibilities of investigators are matters of central importance regardless of accreditation and will be taken up in greater depth as the committee continues its work.

Improving Research Monitoring

Research monitoring has emerged as a major problem, but policies have mainly focused on administrative compliance with federal regulations that emphasize informed consent and prospective review of written protocols. One reason is that the level of administrative compliance is much easier to measure and infractions are thus easier to document. For example, every research protocol must be reviewed, and informed-consent forms and minutes of IRB meetings can reflect specific actions. This creates a trail of documentation that can be audited (or can suggest a remedy when a trail of documentation is not maintained).

Research monitoring, in contrast, is mainly concerned with the prevention of rare bad events. Research monitoring may be the more important function of the system, but effective monitoring is much harder to measure. The current HRPPP system attends to the functional equivalent of maintenance records by documenting informed-consent forms and IRB deliberations, but it appears to be less adept at identifying and investigating serious breaches or systematically detecting danger signals in ongoing research. In most cases, the trigger for an investigation has come from participants who make complaints, research staff who act as whistleblowers, or public media exposure and investigative journalism.[13]

If the oversight processes are working well, serious violations will be rare. Learning from such rare violations, however, is essential to improving the system, and the current system appears to be deficient in this function. The elements of the protection regime most amenable to accreditation, moreover, may not be the ones most likely to first identify serious infractions or problems. The oversight system could, however, become much more systematic about detecting problems by creating feedback mechanisms by which research participants and staff can report problems (and can link those reports to IRBs), by ensuring that means for the identification and reporting of serious and unexpected adverse events are built into the research process, and by strengthening linkages between programs for HRPPP review and programs for investigation of the serious problems that do arise.

The relative roles of institutions conducting research, research sponsors, accreditation bodies, and OHRP and the FDA in investigating violations are not clearly spelled out. Historical cases suggest that research institutions are sometimes delegated primary responsibility for investigation (for example, the University of California at Los Angeles for the Cline case), and at times federal regulatory agencies take the lead (for example, the FDA for the Gelsinger case).

---

[13] The Tuskegee trial, Martin Cline's premature gene therapy experiments, and human radiation experiments were all first reported in the public media, with investigations occurring after public furor. The FDA had begun to investigate the death of Jesse Gelsinger when the case became public, but many of the details about financial conflict of interest and serious underreporting of adverse events became known mainly via investigative journalism. Investigations then followed.

The emergence of accreditation bodies will introduce new organizations with important roles to play in learning from lapses in the system to ensure continuous improvement, making it all the more important to spell out the roles and responsibilities of different parties when serious infractions come to light.

Large multicenter clinical trials now routinely include formal data safety and monitoring boards (DSMBs). DSMBs were initially established to assist research sponsors with analysis of their data, but their importance in assessing risk and monitoring safety has become apparent. Such boards are typically composed of researchers with expertise similar to that of the principal investigators, but they come from independent research institutions and are augmented by statisticians, bioethicists, and sometimes lawyers and consumers. The only personnel requirements for NIH DSMBs are that they include expert clinicians and experts in biometrics or statistics. These monitoring boards receive reports of study outcomes, including both intended effects and adverse events. They pool findings from multiple centers (findings which the individual centers often do not receive and to which only research sponsors would otherwise have access). DSMBs may stop a trial if it appears to be causing harm or if its study objective is met early. A DSMB can also become the locus for receiving reports of mishaps and complaints, as well as adverse events and research outcomes.

NIH has recently mandated that any NIH-sponsored clinical trial have a research monitoring plan and that the plan take into account the level of risk (NIH, 2000). The National Cancer Institute has mandated that any phase III trial (a large trial, typically conducted at many centers, intended to demonstrate the efficacy of an intervention) have a DSMB (NCI, 1999). The inclusion of such boards has been standard practice in most trials sponsored by private industry to test new drugs, devices, or biologics. The Good Clinical Practice portion of the International Conference on Harmonisation guidelines that govern clinical trials has an entire section (section 5.18) devoted to monitoring (International Conference on Harmonisation of Technical Requirements for Registration of Pharmaceuticals for Human Use, 1996, pp. 26–29). The connections between DSMBs and IRBs are not completely consistent, however. Although all DSMBs are accountable to research sponsors for the integrity of the data, their role in ensuring safety and in protecting research participants is less well articulated. They are not always clearly accountable to IRBs, and their responsibilities to research participants or groups representing the interests of research participants are sometimes not explicit.

WILL ACCREDITATION ENHANCE PERFORMANCE?

The interaction between accreditation bodies and the organizations that they accredit can indicate new strategies for improving performance. Over the past three decades the constant lament of dozens of reports from a half dozen knowledgeable commissions has been that the current HRPPP system emphasizes administrative compliance when it would do better to focus on the rights and interests of research participants, the risks that they face, and whether their choices are fully autonomous. Yet, the federal regulations governing the protection of human research subjects have been largely the same for 25 years, and it took a decade to get agreement on the federal Common Rule among 18 agencies. The arduousness of that task has itself become an argument for leaving the regulations intact, but that is a recipe for stagnation in a research enterprise that is rapidly growing and changing. Even an experiment to have a "central IRB" at the National Cancer Institute took 2 years to launch. The federal regulatory system is indeed rigid and focused on documentation rather than performance (see discussion under Applying the Models to Human Research Oversight).

An accreditation process should "emphasize outcomes or performance rather than structure, process, and procedures," and "successful accreditation bodies are flexible, future-oriented, and constantly looking at changes taking place in their fields to make sure the standards and review process are relevant to the needs of the accredited entities" (Hamm, 1997, pp. 72–73). For the first time in decades, the HRPPP system is in flux with the elevation of OHRP out of NIH and a recent shift to an IRB registration process linked to a streamlined assurance process by OHRP (OHRP, 2000b) along the lines of a recommendation by C. K. Gunsalus in a report to NBAC (Gunsalus, forthcoming). These changes were possible without a revamping of federal regulations, but flexibility beyond this will be more difficult to achieve. If a nongovernmental accreditation system could fulfill the promise of flexibility, provide an orientation toward performance, and provide adaptability, it could measurably improve the HRPPP system over time.

In the immediate future, the emphasis on HRPPP accreditation, based on the draft standards and procedures proposed, appears to be bringing existing HRPPPs into compliance with existing federal regulations. The aspiration, however, is higher, and that may be possible, but the problem is difficult. In congressional testimony in 1994, Robyn Nishimi of the Office of Technology Assessment observed:

> The current system, while changing incrementally, has fallen short of implementing, or did not implement at all, recommendations made between 1973 and 1982 by an ad hoc committee of DHEW, a congressional report and two congressionally mandated commissions (Nishimi, 1994, p. 149).

Since Nishimi made that statement, the nation has had reports from ACHRE (ACHRE, 1995), the General Accounting Office (GAO, 1996), and DHHS OIG (DHHS OIG, 1998a,b,c,d,e, 2000a,b,c). NBAC's report on those with mental disabilities and two forthcoming NBAC reports also contain many recommendations that warrant action (NBAC, 1998, forthcoming-a,b). An independent voluntary accreditation system appears to be one element that could improve the system as part of a long-term strategy and, thus, should be pilot tested and evaluated over the next several years.

3

Standards for Accreditation

Any set of standards used by accreditation organizations responsible for the protection of research participants must be flexible enough to be applicable to a variety of institutions yet rigorous enough to ensure that their enactment enhances protection of human research participants. In addition, they must be clearly written, relatively straightforward to execute, consistently applicable, and measurable. These are not easy goals.

In response to a request from the U.S. Department of Health and Human Services (DHHS), the Institute of Medicine was asked to address accreditation standards for human research participant protection programs (HRPPPs). To accomplish this task, the committee reviewed draft versions of proposed standards developed by Public Responsibility in Medicine and Research (PRIM&R) and the National Committee for Quality Assurance (NCQA), as well as the International Conference on Harmonisation Guidelines for Good Clinical Practice (ICH-GCP).

The PRIM&R standards were drafted to be used as measurement criteria for a new voluntary program for research protection. The standards are intended to guide organizations seeking private voluntary accreditation in the assessment of their human research protection programs (HRPPs) and to be used by independent site visitors during the accreditation process.

NCQA is an independent, nonprofit organization under contract with the U.S. Department of Veterans Affairs (VA) to operate an accreditation program to ensure that VA medical centers are complying with VA and other relevant federal regulations designed to protect human participants in research.

ICH-GCP represents an "international ethical and scientific quality standard for designing, conducting, recording, and reporting trials that involve the participation of human subjects" (International Conference on Harmonisation of Technical Requirements for Registration of Pharmaceuticals for Human Use, 1996, p. 1). In addition to being widely accepted in the clinical trials community, the ICH-GCP standards are recognized by the Office for Human Research Protections (OHRP) and included within the Food and Drug Administration (FDA) guidance document for clinical trials. Although these are guidelines for investigators and research sponsors conducting or supporting clinical trials, they specifically address the roles and responsibilities of these parties at a level of detail not found in either the PRIM&R or NCQA standards and are thus directly relevant to the assessment of HRPPPs.

As the committee struggled in a short period of time to develop a "theory" on which the standards for accreditation of HRPPPs could be based, the challenges and perhaps impossibility of developing a "one-size-fits-all" approach became apparent. The three sets of standards were reminders of the vastness of the research enterprise and the distinctive nature of certain types of research and research settings. For example, the PRIM&R standards appear to focus on research conducted in traditional academic health care settings, the NCQA standards encompass research conducted by the VA in its own self-contained health care system, and the ICH-GCP guidelines are specific to investigators and sponsors conducting clinical trials, a specialized type of research with human participants.

Even so, the three distinct research situations described above all pertain to biomedical research environments. As discussed in Chapter 1, this does not adequately represent the multiple contexts in which human research occurs. The breadth of these research contexts creates layers of complexity that are not easily absorbed when a single set of standards is being developed for the assessment of performance. An organization's scope of activities should define which standards apply. Moreover, the accreditation body must consider the degree to which an HRPPP must comply with the standards. That is, must an organization be in full compliance with every standard to become accredited? Or should the organization demonstrate overall compliance with the full set of applicable standards? The answers to these questions might dictate the magnitude and scope of a set of standards and the level of detail that is necessary to support them. If the goal is to develop a single set of standards, such standards must accommodate several types of organizations engaged in the review and conduct of research with human participants.

STANDARDS FOR STANDARDS

At a minimum, standards should address an organization's level of performance in specific areas and, some would argue, not just what the organization is capable of doing but what it actually does (JCAHO, 2000). In theory, standards should set forth maximum achievable performance expectations for activities that affect the protection of human research participants. Perhaps most importantly, they should be based on widely accepted ethical principles that form the norms for research behavior.

In the United States, the principles embodied in *The Belmont Report* have served as the foundation for the ethical requirements in human research (National Commission for the Protection of Human Subjects of Biomedical and Behavioral Research, 1979). The three basic ethical principles in *The Belmont Report* are (1) respect for persons, (2) beneficence, and (3) justice. The first principle, respect for persons, encompasses two ethical concepts: first, "individuals should be treated as autonomous agents" and their decisions respected; and second, "persons with diminished autonomy are entitled to protection" (p. 4). The second principle, beneficence, incorporates the rules of "do no harm" and "maximize possible benefits and minimize possible harms" (p. 4). The third principle, justice, refers to a fair and equitable distribution of benefits and burdens, fair selection of participants, assurance that participants receive what is deserved or due, and ascertainment that equals are treated equally (p. 5). In the United States, these principles strongly influenced the development of federal regulations—in particular, regulations governing research sponsored by the federal government or regulated by the FDA—via the Federal Policy for the Protection of Human Subjects (45 CFR 46, subpart A, also known as the "Common Rule") or parallel FDA regulations (21 CFR 50, 56; international studies of devices are covered by 21 CFR 312.120).

The ethical principles found in *The Belmont Report* are also found in many international documents, including the Declaration of Helsinki and guidelines promulgated by the Council for International Organizations of Medical Sciences, a source on the ethics of international research involving human subjects (CIOMS, 1993; World Medical Association, 2000).

The ethical principles should be accompanied by procedural requirements, which then form the basis of the standards. Thus, standards should have an explicit rationale that is consistent with the goal of protecting individuals or populations that participate in research. The committee's "standards for standards" are contained in two recommendations.

Recommendation 3: Articulate Sound Goals Within Acreditation Standards

The goals of accreditation standards should be to ensure
1. that the proposed research promises to contribute knowledge sufficient to justify research involving human participants;
2. independent review of research by a board knowledgeable about protection standards and the fields of research being reviewed;

3. that the perspectives of participants are represented on institutional review boards (IRBs), on research monitoring bodies, and throughout the research oversight system;

4. that IRB members do not review protocols with which they have financial or nonfinancial conflicts of interest;[1]

5. that investigator and institutional conflicts of interest, both financial and nonfinancial, are disclosed to IRBs and participants and are managed responsibly by research institutions;

6. a review process that balances risks and potential benefits, keeps risks to the minimum necessary, and monitors research on a continuing basis;

7. that an effective process for obtaining voluntary informed consent of participants is in place;

8. that policies and procedures to assess the quality of HRPPP operations, enhance accountability, and improve performance are in place;

9. there is fairness in the recruitment and selection of participants;

10. that the privacy and confidentiality of research participants are protected; and

11. that the HRPPP is transparent so that participants can judge the research process to be trustworthy.

Recommendation 4: Establish Flexible, Ethics-Based, and Meaningful Standards

Accreditation standards should meet the following minimal criteria:

1. They should be based on sound and widely accepted ethical principles.[2]

---

[1] The committee does not mean that any member who could have a conflict with any conceivable protocol coming to an IRB for review should be excluded from service on an IRB but, rather, that the individual should recuse himself or herself from reviewing such protocols.

[2] The principles laid out in *The Belmont Report* are one foundation (National Commission for the Protection of Human Subjects of Biomedical and Behavioral Research, 1979). Accreditation standards, however, should also incorporate the recommendations of the President's Commission for the Study of Ethical Problems in Medicine and Biomedical and Behavioral Research (President's Commission, 1981, 1983), the recommendations of the Advisory Committee for Human Radiation Experiments (ACHRE, 1995), recommendations presented in reports of the National Bioethics Advisory Commission (NBAC, 1997, 1998, 1999a,b, forthcoming-a,b), the recommendations of the Office of the Inspector General of DHHS (DHHS OIG, 1998b, 2000b), and the recommendations of the General Accounting Office (GAO, 1996). In addition, recommendations from reports and declarations of private bodies and independent scholars should be incorporated. This presupposes that an advisory apparatus is available to cull this literature.

2. They should be flexible and adapted to different kinds of research and different research institutions.

3. They should encourage accredited organizations to shift from a culture that relies on external compliance checks to a culture that puts safety and voluntary participation foremost.

4. They should facilitate compliance with federal regulations but should aim to move an organization toward having stronger protection of human research participants.

5. To the extent possible, they should focus on the use of meaningful measures of how well the rights and interests of research participants are being protected rather than simple determination of whether informed-consent statements have been signed or IRB meetings were duly constituted.

Measurement of an organization's compliance with the procedural requirements set forth by standards serves as a proxy for ascertainment of the organization's level of compliance with the ethical principles that underlie the standards.

In its early discussions, the committee noted that beyond the primary aspiration of protecting those who participate in research, institutions seeking accreditation will be motivated by other aims as well, for example, enhancing the qualities and reputations of their research programs (and, as a result, potentially improving their financial status or prestige), attracting faculty and students to their graduate research training programs, and facilitating the recruitment of individuals as research participants. A successful system of accreditation must offer incentives for participation, such as enhancing the likelihood that a program in compliance with the standards will attract these resources. In addition, a successful accreditation system must have realistic and enforceable mechanisms by which to deter noncompliance with the standards (e.g., suspension from the program or loss of accreditation).

DEVELOPING MEASURES TO ACCOMPANY STANDARDS

Standards must be developed with consideration of the measures that will be used to evaluate an organization's level of compliance. The processes of developing standards and designing a set of tools that can be used to measure compliance (i.e., accreditation) cannot generally be uncoupled. The measures must address areas in which performance is likely to have a significant impact on the protection of human research populations. In addition, they must be precisely defined and specified, that is, standardized with explicit predefined requirements for data collection and for calculation of the value of the measure or the score for the measure. Furthermore, for the purpose of accreditation, there must be documentation for the measure that includes defined data elements, corresponding data sources, and allowable values. Such measures must be reliable—that is, the measurement should be able to identify consistently the events that it was designed to identify across multiple HRPPPs over time—and they must be valid, that is, they must capture what they were intended to measure.

The tools used to measure compliance with standards should be easily interpreted by those who use the resulting data, including accreditors, research participants, and those conducting or overseeing the research. Finally, determinations of the levels of compliance with the standards must be based on data. HRPPPs seeking accreditation will be required to provide evidence of compliance. This evidence must be supported by a reasonable data collection effort. In the development of standards, accreditation bodies must be mindful of the availability and accessibility of the required data elements and the effort and cost of abstracting and collecting data.

In general, standards should help HRPPPs and accreditation bodies identify exemplary performance and best practices, thus serving as a benchmarking service for the organizations seeking accreditation. In addition, ideal standards would provide the content for publicly available comparative reports on the performance of the accredited organization.

This view of accreditation standards is reflected in *Understanding Accreditation* (Young et al., 1983), which notes four trends in the accreditation process: (1) it has moved from a more quantitative to a more qualitative system of assessment, with more general rather than specific standards; (2) it has placed less emphasis on making institutions look alike and more emphasis on a stance of recognizing and encouraging individuality; (3) it has evolved from a system based more on external review to a system of self-evaluation and self-regulation; and (4) it has moved from a focus on the institution to a focus on encouraging and assisting the organization in its efforts to improve quality.

In this light, standards should describe important functions related to the protection of research participants, and they should be framed as performance objectives that are unlikely to change substantially over time. Because standards aim to improve outcomes, they should place minimal emphasis on how to achieve these objectives. In addition any set of standards should make clear which standards are cores, that is, those that must be applied across programs and that are essential to an HRPPP. Some standards, such as those that directly relate to the protection of human research participants, should carry more weight than others. It is especially important that clear measurement tools be available for core standards and that guidance on how the measurement will be interpreted is available.

NEED FOR STANDARDS TO ENCOMPASS
MULTIPLE RESEARCH SETTINGS AND METHODS

Recommendation 5: Accommodate Distinct Research Methods and Models Within Accreditation Programs

The accreditation process should accommodate other research organizations in addition to the tradtional models provided by academic health centers and VA facilities. The accreditation process should also cover research other than clinical research.

Standards must accommodate the distinct natures of several types of organizations, including research institutions, educational institutions, independent IRBs, academic medical centers, nongovernmental organizations, and private interests. A set of standards can make clear the scope of institutions to which they apply in several ways: (1) state explicitly in the preamble the intended focus of the standards; (2) include flexible language, such as "where applicable" or "as appropriate" to certain standards so that institutions not engaged in particular activities (e.g., nonmedical, low-risk research) could be exempt from certain standards (e.g., reporting of adverse events); or (3) organize the standards so that institutions and accreditation bodies can quickly ascertain which sections apply to them and which ones do not.

If standards were structured in a manner that requires the existence of a single entity with exclusive authority over all parties involved in the research process, then the three requirements listed above would not apply. It must be recognized, however, that certain organizations, such as independent IRBs and some private sponsors of research, would then not be eligible for accreditation. This would be an unfortunate consequence, as it would exclude organizations that play an increasing role in the research enterprise.

Accreditation of an independent IRB, for example, might use only the subset of standards pertinent to IRBs, but doing so would also require formal assurance regarding the functions covered by proposed standards that pertain to investigators, research institutions, and research participants, as well as standards that pertain to sponsors but that are not yet incorporated into NCQA or PRIM&R standards (but covered by ICH-GCP guidelines) (see discussion below). Another approach would be to accredit the organization that directly controls all the relevant elements of an HRPPP (e.g., a contract research organization that has a formal agreement with an independent IRB to review all its protocols, the research unit of a private firm, the unit of a federal agency that performs research, or a clinical trials cooperative group). One of the virtues of a nongovernmental voluntary accreditation process is its flexibility, and nongovernmental accreditation bodies should not find it difficult to accommodate disparate organizational structures. It is not yet clear, however, how the current proposed standards or accreditation processes would do so.

Although there is a natural tendency to develop standards and review procedures around a specific model, accommodation of innovative or unique organizations is central, and although "basing development on a commonly accepted template may benefit the accrediting organization, there is a danger that innovative structures or processes undergoing accreditation will encounter additional challenges or problems in the review process" (Hamm, 1997, p. 31).

In addition to accommodating distinct types of research infrastructures, the language of standards should acknowledge that even though the principles that underlie them apply to all human research, the criteria and mechanisms for review must be adaptable and must be based on the nature of the research being conducted and the context within which the research is to be performed. The committee heard strong, consistent comments that the proposed standards (in this case, those of PRIM&R) do not fully recognize either the diversity of institutions or the full range of research (AAU, COGR, NASULGC, 2001; Kulakowski, 2001; Ryan, 2001). The standards proposed by NCQA under contract with the VA, however, are necessarily limited in scope to VA facilities. Although the committee believes that the same principles for protection of the rights and interests of research participants apply to all research—for example, biomedical, behavioral and social, public health, and outcomes research—it is likely that the processes needed to comply with the standards will differ depending on the nature of the research. Thus, it is an open question whether the best accreditation strategy would be to use one set of operational standards for all research. That might well prove viable, but it also might prove better to encourage the evolution of different specific standards for different kinds of research institutions.

Those in the best position to make this determination will be organizations devising the nongovernmental accreditation processes, not this committee or the federal government. Whether to develop one set of standards or a few sets of standards specific to a few different classes of research organizations should not be decided by fiat but should be decided in light of experience gained through pilot accreditation programs that include medical and nonmedical sites.

Accreditation pilot programs can begin by focusing on the research institutions for which they were designed, but they might evolve in many different ways. In the future, there could be one or a few accreditation bodies and one or a few sets of accreditation standards, and many different kinds of organizations will certainly be involved in research with human participants.

RELATION OF THE STANDARDS TO THE
EXISTING REGULATORY REQUIREMENTS

Recommendation 6: Base Standards on Existing Regulations

Accreditation standards should start from federal regulations for the protection of human research participants but should augment those regulations. The process should be iterative and continual, with evolution of both accreditation standards and the operations of accredited organizations, creating incentives for accredited organizations to improve.

Institutions that receive federal funds, that hold an assurance from OHRP, or that seek FDA approval must comply with the Common Rule or parallel FDA regulations. Therefore, it is important that any standards be considered in relation to the regulatory requirements; that is, are they consistent, supplemental, or contradictory? Many commentators at the committee's public forum, as well as committee members themselves, expressed concern that new standards for accreditation could impose another layer of bureaucracy on a system that is already sagging under the weight of paperwork, but would add little to the protection of human research participants (AAPP, 2001; Cornblath, 2001; Oakes, 2001).

Three issues to be considered in this context: (1) If the standards are identical to federal regulatory standards, both the institution and the accreditor are performing redundant tasks (presumably largely paperwork, assuming that the institution is already in compliance with the federal regulations) unless some simple means is found for the certification of compliance; (2) If the standards are inconsistent with federal regulations, confusion is likely to result; (3) If the standards are more demanding than federal regulations, a question must be raised: are the additional expectations likely to strengthen protections at a reasonable cost?

Accreditation standards should start from the base of regulations governing research with humans. These regulations, in turn, are based on a set of principles for the ethical conduct of research (see Recommendation 4). By the use of standards that emphasize processes of continuous quality improvement instead of an exclusive focus on regulatory compliance (see below), the way may be open to the development of future standards that center on HRPPP performance, in addition to the current focus on documentation. For example, an HRPPP that demonstrates that it can ensure informed consent because it has data showing that participants understand the protocols in which they are enrolled, could begin to supplant or augment paper audits of signed informed-consent forms. This strategy therefore has the potential to introduce the desired flexibility and focus on outcomes into the oversight system. Furthermore, this goal that standards continuously evolve supports the committee's recommendation (Recommendation 2) that HRPPP accreditation bodies be nongovernmental organizations, as the federal regulatory process does not possess the sensitivity and responsiveness to maintain pace with opportunities for improvement.

STANDARDS FOR QUALITY IMPROVEMENT AND SELF-STUDY

Recommendation 7: Incorporate Continuous Quality Improvement Mechanisms into Standards

Accreditation organizations should emphasize the process of self-study, evaluation, and continuous quality improvement among applicants. They should move beyond documentation of informed consent and protocol review, which, although essential, do not of themselves protect the rights and interests of research participants.

Standards provide an HRPPP with the opportunity for benchmarking, a continuous, systematic process used to make improvements. By periodically examining activities, policies, procedures, support functions, organizational performance, and the status of data collection and processing, an HRPPP can develop an approach to quality improvement. A sound system of self-assessment can identify the best practices in an organization and target areas in need of improvement. Compliance with regulatory requirements, in contrast, provides an important but irregular approach to ensuring that protections are in place. Thus, standards not only provide the basis for a system of self-study and improvement but also should incorporate the expectation of such a quality improvement system. This is not to say that self-study alone is sufficient. To maintain the integrity of the accreditation process, an HRPPP must conduct self-study as well as be subjected to external review (whether by an accreditation body or a regulatory agency).

Standards should aim to improve outcomes and should not overly prescribe how to achieve the specified objectives. Rather, they should focus on the core standards that apply across programs and that are essential to a quality HRPPP. Current proposed standards generally reinforce the documentation practices required by federal regulations but do not yet go beyond the regulations. In general, both entities seeking accreditation and accreditation bodies should identify exemplary performance and best practices, providing benchmarks for the research community at large and making information on organization performance openly available to the public and policy makers. In this way, for example, an HRPPP demonstrating a particularly reliable system for the monitoring of participant safety or the reporting of problems in ongoing research, might have an advantage over nonaccredited competitors in seeking support from sponsors or having access to participants, researchers, or students.

NEED FOR STANDARDS TO ENHANCE THE ROLE
OF RESEARCH PARTICIPANTS

Recommendation 8: Directly Involve Research Participants in Accreditation Programs and HRPPPs

The formulation of accreditation standards, the accreditation process, and HRPPP operations should directly involve research participants.[3]

Current regulations lay a foundation for and even invite stronger involvement of those representing the interests of those participating in research. Yet, some "noninstitutional" members of IRBs have little experience as participants in research; they may be independent of the institution, but it does not follow that they represent the perspective of research participants. The regulations are necessarily nonspecific about the involvement of research participants in the review process and set a low standard for qualification. When HRPPPs are regularly judging the benefits and risks of studies that involve particular populations, there should be evidence that the review process directly involved those who genuinely understand and represent the perspective of those populations. This requirement could be incorporated into accreditation standards.

Practices regarding membership on data safety and monitoring boards (DSMBs) are even more diverse. The only stipulated expertise on DSMBs is technical: a clinician familiar with the medical aspects and a statistician familiar with data analysis. In instances in which they attend explicitly to safety and the ethical conduct of research, DSMBs are more apt to include a bioethicist or a lawyer than someone who brings the perspective of research participants. Accreditation standards—and even more so, the guidance documents that accompany them by giving examples of good practices—can improve the HRPPP system to ensure stronger representation of the interests of the research participants.

Given the primacy of the concepts of autonomy in research ethics and the training of IRB members, the relative lack of attention to standards and measures that would systematically cultivate these concepts in both the PRIM&R and NCQA proposed standards is somewhat surprising (see the discussion in the What's Missing section below). Several measures can be taken to bolster these concepts to improve the ethical conduct of research involving human participants. IRBs, DSMBs, research design teams, and merit review committees should increase their level of attention to the involvement of research participants or those who genuinely represent participants' perspectives in the design, selection, review, and monitoring of research involving human participants. In

---

[3] By "participants," the committee refers to those whose background and expertise are credible to a lay constituency external to the research institution and who are knowledgeable about the research process and research protections. The term is further defined in Chapter 1.

addition to including more research participants in the review and oversight process, standards could require institutions to engage in additional activities to improve the process for research participant involvement in the system.

Institutions that conduct research can create ombudsman programs, particularly for studies that may cause confusion among participants or that entail significant risks. The ombudsman can receive information that participants have about the studies in which they are involved (or in which they are contemplating participation). The same mechanism can be used by research staff or other employees of the research institution who may be uncomfortable with how a study is being conducted, if confidentiality is ensured and anti-retaliation policies are clear (and credible) for prospective whistle blowers.

IRBs can ensure safe, confidential, and reliable channels for the reporting of problems. The channels either can be linked to ombudsman programs or can be independent of them (e.g., having assigned staff and formal policies to encourage such reporting).

Investigators (or IRBs) can test whether participants' consent is well informed by empirically testing it and following up when necessary. Several methods have been studied and reported in the scant empirical literature on research ethics (Sugarman, 2000). One method is to use consent monitors—that is, staff who interview participants after the participants have given their consent to participate in a study to see if they understood the study, the risks and potential benefits, and their ability to leave the study at any time. This option is expensive and time-consuming and cannot be routine, but it could be used for particularly confusing or risky studies and could be done as a general sampling technique or research strategy to guide IRBs about the research that they review.

Likewise, consumer organizations can address the need for informed participant involvement by training representatives to participate directly in the design, review, and monitoring of research.[4]

Private organizations of citizens have long been a potent force in U.S. research policy. Hundreds of private voluntary health organizations are directly involved in advocacy for health research, and they often play decisive roles in decisions about research budgets and priorities, which is perhaps their best-known function. Their concerns do not stop at funding, however, but extend to the ethical conduct of research not only to encourage high-quality research to meet participants' health needs but also to protect the perspective of their constituents. Where the infrastructure already exists, HRPPPs merely need to solicit input more systematically and ensure that consumer groups are well represented on IRBs, DSMBs, and other design and oversight bodies. The constituencies for

---

[4] The National Breast Cancer Coalition, for example, has Project LEAD (Leadership, Education and Advocacy Development) that trains advocates to serve on research review and advisory panels, and the National Alliance for the Mentally Ill has a program that trains members to serve on IRBs.

some conditions, however, are less well organized and may require funding from research sponsors, both public and private, to build the capacity for research oversight.

Accreditation programs can systematically solicit desired outcomes from research participants. In his book on accreditation, Michael Hamm (Hamm, 1997) alluded several times to the desirability of having a focus on outcomes and performance rather than process and structure. The outcomes most desired in an HRPPP are an independent review of risks and benefits and a genuine process of informed consent. Participants are directly relevant to the informed-consent process in particular. The literature on empirical studies of the informed-consent process suggests that investigators often do not know what participants hear, and investigators are poor judges of what participants understand.

Those who develop accreditation standards would do well to directly involve focus groups, consent monitors, and participant representatives (e.g., those who themselves have been involved in past studies or who are educated about the research process and ethical standards but who are also familiar with the interests of a constituency) in specifying the desired outcomes to be incorporated into accreditation standards. Accreditation bodies could invite private voluntary health organizations and other organizations representing research participants[5] to help formulate points to be considered in the development of accreditation standards and modification of the standards as they evolve.

NEED FOR STANDARDS REGARDING ROLES AND RESPONSIBILITIES OF RESEARCH SPONSORS

Neither the PRIM&R nor the NCQA draft standards address standards for sponsors. The PRIM&R document defines sponsor as, "Any entity that provides funds or other resources to support the research. This entity could be a federal agency, corporation, foundation, institution or an individual" (see Appendix B, Glossary). It is noteworthy that in most cases it will not be the sponsor that is seeking accreditation as an HRPPP. However, there will be some examples in which the research institution that conducts and reviews the studies is also paying for a particular research project. In addition, when the sponsor is a federal agency, the assurance process results in an agreement between the sponsor and the research institution that federal regulatory requirements will be met.

The committee recognizes that it would be difficult to incorporate such standards into the accreditation programs for HRPPPs; however, it believes that such standards should exist. These standards would provide research institutions, investigators, and IRBs with a set of expectations that should be met when

---

[5] For research not on a particular medical condition, the constituency may be, for example, veterans at VA facilities or representatives of the general public familiar with research methods and ethical canons for general population studies.

they review research protocols sponsored by external sources. The ICH-GCP guidelines provide a useful starting point, although they are narrowly focused on clinical trials.

Accreditation of HRPPPs could leave the responsibilities of research sponsors outside the accreditation framework but not necessarily outside the scope of regulation by the FDA or OHRP. FDA regulations, for example, place the mantle of responsibility for the ethical conduct of research on sponsors, and the ICH-GCP guidelines have a section devoted to sponsor responsibilities. For clinical trials of drugs, devices, and other products subject to FDA regulation, FDA staff would continue to hold sponsors accountable by site visits, audits, investigation, enforcement, and other activities already performed by agency staff. Sponsors may continue to be liable if they do not make reasonable efforts to determine whether participant protection systems are in place at research institutions where they are conducting research. Similarly, accreditation bodies should develop standards by which HRPPPs should determine the acceptability of funding from a given source.

The other alternative is to consider the research units within sponsoring organizations as the logical unit for accreditation, but this would require an entirely new framework and would entail accreditation of dozens of pharmaceutical firms, hundreds of biotechnology firms, and many federal agencies that directly sponsor research. This framework diverges sharply from the accreditation models proposed to the committee.

To address the role of sponsors, standards could include the following:

• The sponsor is responsible, where applicable, for implementing and maintaining quality assurance and control systems to ensure that studies are generated and documented in compliance with the protocol and applicable regulatory requirements.

• The sponsor should ensure that the peer review and design components of funded protocols meet the highest standards and that efforts are made to use the least number of participants possible while maintaining statistical relevance.

• The sponsor should ensure that the research team is appropriately trained and qualified to conduct the research.

• The sponsor should permit disclosure of the financial interests that investigators have in a research project as a result of the funding received for that project.

• The sponsor is responsible for reporting to all concerned investigators, institutions, and regulatory authorities any adverse events resulting from research studies.

REVIEW OF AVAILABLE DRAFT STANDARDS

The two draft sets of standards reviewed by the committee represent an initial step in constructing an accreditation system. However, standards are only as good as the guidelines and measures used to assess compliance with them. Thus, many questions that arise from review of the drafts might be resolved only when they are considered in the context of the guidelines that will accompany them and experience gained through pilot testing.

In reviewing the PRIM&R and NCQA standards the committee found it useful to assess them according to the following general criteria: (1) their scope and focus; (2) their relationship to the existing regulatory standards; and (3) the extent to which the standards can be consistently implemented, measured, and enforced, as well as their inclusion of various key elements (see Table 3-1).

In addition to the two sets of proposed accreditation standards examined, the committee considered the ICH-GCP guidelines on the basis of their inclusion of widely accepted guidelines (internationally and domestically) for research sponsors and investigators involved in clinical trials.

Scope and Focus of the Standards

PRIM&R Standards

The PRIM&R standards (Appendix B) appropriately imply that the ethical principles described in *The Belmont Report* (National Commission for the Protection of Human Subjects of Biomedical and Behavioral Research, 1979) should serve as the fundamental inspiration for institutions seeking to promote research while protecting those who participate in it. However, they appear to be written mainly with academic medical centers that house one or more IRBs in mind. The PRIM&R document states that accreditation applies to the human research protection program (HRPP). Outside traditional academic health centers, it is not clear what entity would be responsible for the HRPP and hence for seeking accreditation.

One test of the broader utility of the PRIM&R standards (and those of NCQA) is whether they could be easily applied in other research settings, such as private industry, institutions that rely on independent IRBs, survey organizations, community hospitals, and teaching institutions with largely undergraduate student populations, or even in instances of multisite trials or collaborative IRB review. As discussed earlier in this chapter, all accreditation programs must be adaptable to a broad range of research environments, methods, and review mechanisms (Recommendation 5).

An additional observation relates to the apparent focus on the IRB as the central arbiter of the protection of human participants. If, in fact, the activities surrounding the protection of human participants in research are evolving into a system, then this focus seems too narrow. Although the standards mention the

TABLE 3-1 Elements in Three Sets of Standards and Guidelines

Key Elements	Organization Developing the Standard or Guideline		
	PRIM&R	NCQA	ICH
Intended use	Standards	Standards	Guidelines
Targeted sites or bodies	Research institutions (U.S.)	VA facilities	Organizations conducting clinical trials of drugs
Foundational principles	The Belmont Report[a]	The Belmont Report	Declaration of Helsinki[b]
Regulatory relevance	Implied	45 CFR 46, 21 CFR 50 and 56, and VA regulations are the starting points (cross-referenced)	Drug approval regulations in the European Union, Japan, and the United States
Components affected	• Organizations • IRBs • Investigators and other personnel	• HRPPs • Institutions • IRBs • Investigators	• IRBs or ethics review committee • Investigators • Sponsors
Link to quality improvement program?	No	Yes	No
Standards for participant involvement (beyond consent)?	No	No	No
Standards for sponsors?	No	No[c]	Yes
Standards for monitoring?	Limited, one mention in one documentation standard	Yes	Yes

Specific guidance for interpreting standards?	No	Yes	Yes
Data source identified?	For some documentation standards	Yes	Yes
Methods for measuring provided?	No, except documentation standards	Yes	Partial
Thresholds established for compliance?	No	Yes	No
Appeals process	No	Yes	Yes

[a]National Commission for the Protection of Human Subjects of Biomedical and Behavioral Research (1979).

[b]World Medical Association (1964).

[c]NCQA standards are written for research conducted in VA facilities. For research conducted at VA facilities but sponsored by external sources (e.g., National Institutes of Health; the U.S. Department of Defense; or pharmaceutical device, or biotechnology firms), additional sponsor provisions, such as written agreement to abide by ICH-GCP guidelines, would be needed.

roles and responsibilities of investigators and the "organization" (e.g., institutional officials, administrative offices, personnel, existing compliance programs, or oversight mechanisms), there is far less attention to these parties than to IRBs, and little to no mention is made of the roles and responsibilities of research sponsors, despite the central role that sponsors play in much of the privately funded research.

NCQA Standards

The standards developed for the VA by NCQA (Appendix C) are distinct in that they are applicable to a defined system. The VA conducts biomedical, health services, and rehabilitation research to improve the health care delivered to the nation's veterans. The VA has developed policies, consistent with the Common Rule and FDA regulations, to safeguard human participants in research and has established the Office of Research Compliance and Assurance (ORCA) to support the field operations in protecting human participants and to assess their compliance with regulations that protect human research participants. The standards will be applied to VA hospitals and VA employees. In that sense, the standards do not face the same level of complexity in the field as the proposed PRIM&R standards do. Nonetheless, they appear to be potentially applicable, with some additions and modifications, to research conducted in other, non-VA, nonmedical settings (see Table 3-1).

The draft NCQA standards are notable in several respects. First, they are not overly prescriptive, although they do begin (as do the PRIM&R standards) from the base of federal regulations (see below). Second, the NCQA standards specifically rely on institutional policies and procedures as the methods by which standards are met. The explicit "data source" for several of the standards is the policies and procedures documentation on file at the institution or the quality improvement document maintained by the institution (see Recommendation 7). This is noteworthy because although the standards will apply to a system that is far more homogeneous than the general research environment, they allow variations in procedures, perhaps recognizing that even within the VA health care system there will be institutional variations.

Third, the standards provide thresholds for compliance in each core area: the IRB, informed consent, institutional accountability, privacy and confidentiality, recruitment and subject selection, and risks and benefits. Thus, to receive full compliance with a requirement, a site must achieve compliance with specified "critical elements." The site may still receive partial compliance with the requirement if those elements are not met[6] (see previous discussion in the section Developing Measures to Accompany Standards).

---

[6] For more information on this process, see http://www.ncqa.org/Pages/Programs/QSG/vastandards.htm.

Relation to Existing Regulatory Requirements

As suggested in Recommendation 6, both the PRIM&R and the NCQA draft standards use the current regulatory standards as the "starting point" for the development of their accreditation programs (Chodosh, 2000; Goldschmidt, 2001). In fact, Standards 1.2 and 1.3 in the PRIM&R standards state that "the organization must uphold ethical principles underlying the protection of individuals studied in research" and that "the organization must assure compliance with applicable legal requirements, including state and local laws" (see Appendix B). However, in the PRIM&R document, there are some instances in which consistency with the federal regulations could be more explicit and concise, such as the reporting of adverse events to the National Institutes of Health, research sponsors, the FDA, IRBs, and institutional biosafety committees. The relationship of the standards to additional regulatory requirements, such as DSMBs and emerging medical privacy regulations, should be considered and made clear.

A notable aspect of the NCQA standards is that they cross-reference the federal regulations. This is a useful approach and one that will be welcomed by administrators facing competing guidelines, regulations, and standards. In addition, because they rely on the regulations to establish which research must be reviewed by an IRB and which research requires retrieval of informed consent, they provide the flexibility that is needed to exclude some types of minimal-risk research from full review and also possibly the requirement to obtain informed consent.

Extent to Which the Standards Can Be Implemented, Measured, and Enforced

To be measurable, there must be some objective means through which the extent to which a program is in compliance with accreditation standards can be gauged. Put another way, if an institution was denied accreditation or had its accreditation revoked, are the standards sufficiently well defined and consistently applied that the accreditor could defend its decision in court? The need for objective measurement tools is critical to ensuring consistency and diminishing arbitrary subjectivity in the accreditation system. What is considered independent and credible in one institution might not be considered so in another.

In the material provided by PRIM&R, some of the standards seem largely hortatory.[7] Some committee members found it difficult to envision how these standards could be implemented, measured, or enforced (except perhaps retrospectively, after egregious noncompliance). For instance, the language directed toward investigators in Standard 3.1 and 3.2 (Appendix B) is very important, as investigator conduct is essential to the realization of ethical research. It is not clear, however, how one would ensure in an objective way that investigators are

---

[7] For example, Standards 1.1, 1.7, 3.1, and 3.2 (Appendix B). Documentation standards are more specific, but many other standards are similarly hortatory.

meeting the PRIM&R standards. Data collection from even a sample of investigators at an accreditation site would be overwhelming, and sample bias would be a very serious concern. The committee therefore had a difficult time conceiving of how these standards could be effectively enforced, even if a useful measurement approach could be devised.

On the other hand, several standards do indeed seem measurable but appear to depend on the production or appropriate filing of pieces of paper (or other bits of data) and may have little to do with the quality of research or protecting the rights and interests of participants. For example, standards for IRB minutes and record keeping are fairly prescriptive and provide some measure of activity for individuals inspecting or accrediting a site. Although the ability to keep accurate records is necessary, it is insufficient to guarantee an effective human research protection program.

Similarly, the NCQA standards also possess a reliance on documentation already called for in federal regulations. However, the NCQA program is based on the assumption that an institutional quality improvement program exists at the organization seeking accreditation (in this case VA facilities). The quality improvement documentation is an important source of data for the accreditation body, serving as a measure of performance at a particular point in time but also as a measure of change over time. This strategy provides the opportunity within the NCQA HRPP accreditation standards to become less reliant on documentation and more reliant on performance (Recommendation 7).

The NCQA standards clearly articulate the data source and measurement method to be used by the accreditation organization. As noted above, this is a real strength because clear indications of the data source to be tapped and an unambiguous method for the measurement of compliance with the standards must be developed in conjunction with the standards if they are to be workable.

In contrast, evaluation of the level of compliance with the PRIM&R standards has not been thoroughly described in the materials reviewed by the committee. It is not enough for the institution to just have policies. It must also follow them. In the absence of clear guidance on how outcomes should be measured, determination of whether an institution meets these standards could be daunting for both accreditors and the organizations that they are accrediting.

What Is Missing

The committee identified a few topics that do not appear to be explicitly included in the current drafts of the PRIM&R and the NCQA standards. Both lack standards for improving participant involvement in the local research review and decision-making processes. There is little to no mention of the rights and responsibilities of research participants or the need for subject participation in the functions of the HRPP (except for those that are required by regulation). In addition, the standards might better address some procedural approaches to the inclusion of research participants in the HRPP (see discussion following Recommendation 8). However, members of the Program Advisory Committee for the NCQA accreditation system will be selected from research stakeholder groups, including participant advocates, and will consider programmatic issues to advise the Program Accreditation Committee (the decision-making group for this program).

As mentioned earlier, the roles and responsibilities of research sponsors are important omissions from both sets of standards that should be addressed. In the case of the NCQA draft standards, it is possible that VA headquarters, through ORCA, is developing standard operating procedures that establish standards when the VA is the sole sponsor. However, for externally sponsored research conducted at VA facilities, HRPP standards or assurance that sponsors are abiding by ICH-GCP or other accepted external standards is needed.

INTERNATIONAL CONFERENCE ON HARMONISATION GUIDELINE FOR GOOD CLINICAL PRACTICE

The ICH-GCP was developed as a handbook for researchers conducting clinical trials, particularly drug trials conducted by sponsors and researchers from more than one country (International Conference on Harmonisation of Technical Requirements for Registration of Pharmaceuticals for Human Use, 1996, 1997). Although the guidelines presented in the ICH-GCP are not actually standards, they provide a clear and explicit set of best practices for those conducting clinical trials (see Box 3-1). The committee looked to the ICH-GCP because it includes defined goals for sponsors and investigators. However, it does not address, per se, the institutions or the setting in which the research will be conducted. As such, the ICH-GCP is "portable" and is therefore an important contribution to enhancing the protection of research participants, wherever the clinical trial is conducted. Aspects of the ICH-GCP serve as clearly delineated models for investigator and sponsor behavior, and, thus, the responsibilities contained within these models should be included in the development of guidelines for HRPPPs. The ideals or norms that the document espouses, however, would need to be translated into standards, and such standards would have to be applicable beyond clinical trials and biomedical research methods.

RECOMMENDATION FOR INITIAL STANDARDS TO
BEGIN PILOT TESTING

Recommendation 9: Use Modified NCQA Standards to Initiate Pilot Programs

Pilot accreditation programs should start from the accreditation standards and processes proposed by NCQA for VA facilities, as adapted for use in other organizational contexts. In expanding the draft NCQA accreditation standards for use beyond VA facilities, the standards should be strengthened in six specific ways as pilot testing commences.

The PRIM&R standards were prepared for a broad set of potential applicant organizations, which would include but not be restricted to academic health centers. The NCQA standards were explicitly prepared for accreditation of VA medical facilities. In this instance, the applicant pool is defined, and, in fact, pilot tests that will use those standards are being planned as this report goes to press.

As noted throughout this discussion of report recommendations, the committee regards the NCQA standards as an excellent starting point for accreditation of VA facilities. The committee recommends, however, that the NCQA standards be strengthened in six areas, to specify (1) how investigators will be reviewed beyond the review of the protocols that they submit for IRB approval;[8] (2) whether and how research sponsors will be assessed in the accreditation process;[9] (3) how participants will be involved in setting standards and accrediting HRPPPs;[10]

---

[8] For research programs involving only a small set of investigators, accreditors might contact all of them; for most programs, however, accreditors would need to sample investigators in a way that is independent of control by the IRB or the institution's research administration. How to do this will likely vary by institution and will have to be specified in advance by the accreditation body. The sampling procedure is likely to evolve during the pilot testing phase.

[9] Some organizations do little or no externally sponsored research so they would be exempt from this aspect of accreditation review. Organizations that do sponsored research will vary widely in the number of protocols and the kinds and numbers of sponsors. For programs with extensive externally sponsored research portfolios, accreditation bodies will need to develop sampling methods that are credible and independent of the organization's IRBs and research administration. Standards for this aspect of review could initially start from the ICH-GCP guidelines noted in Table 3.1.

[10] Accreditation bodies will need to develop methods to sample participants in a manner that is credible and independent of IRBs and research administrators of the organizations seeking accreditation. Participants were not surveyed in the 1998 survey of IRBs and investigators commissioned by National Institutes of Health (Bell et al., 1998), yet the committee believes that participant perspectives are essential to judging whether an HRPPP is operating effectively.

BOX 3-1 The International Conference on Harmonisation of Technical Requirements for Registration of Pharmaceuticals for Human Use

The International Conference on Harmonisation of Technical Requirements for Registration of Pharmaceuticals for Human Use is a project that brings together the regulatory authorities of Europe, Japan, and the United States and experts from the pharmaceutical industry in the three regions to discuss scientific and technical aspects of product registration (or, in the United States, approval for marketing).

The purpose is to make recommendations on ways to achieve greater harmonization in the interpretation and application of technical guidelines and requirements for product registration to reduce or obviate the need to duplicate tests carried out during the research and development process for new medicines. The objectives of such harmonization are the more economical use of human, animal, and material resources and the elimination of unnecessary delay in the global development and availability of new medicines while maintaining safeguards on quality, safety and efficacy, and regulatory obligations to protect public health.

The Guideline for Good Clinical Practice is an international ethical and scientific quality standard for the design, conduct, recording, and reporting of trials that involve the participation of human subjects. Compliance with this standard provides public assurance that the rights, safety, and well-being of trial subjects are protected, consistent with the principles that have their origin in the Declaration of Helsinki, and that the clinical trial data are credible.

The objective of the International Conference on Harmonisation Guideline for Good Clinical Practice (ICH-GCP) is to provide a unified standard by which the European Union, Japan, and the United States can facilitate the mutual acceptance of clinical data by their respective regulatory authorities.

The guideline was developed with consideration of the current good clinical practices of the European Union, Japan, and the United States, as well as those of Australia, Canada, the Nordic countries, and the World Health Organization.

Investigators should follow this guideline when they are generating clinical trial data that are intended to be submitted to regulatory authorities. The principles established in ICH-GCP may also be applied to other clinical investigations that may have an impact on the safety and well-being of human subjects.

SOURCE: http://www.ifpma.org/ich5.html.

(4) how oversight mechanisms can ensure participants' safety in ongoing research;[11] (5) the steps that research institutions and their leadership can take to cultivate a culture that puts the safety and interests of research participants foremost;[12] and (6) mechanisms by which research institutions and, where applicable, research sponsors can be held accountable for ensuring sufficient funding, structural support, and professional rewards for HRPPPs.[13]

The NCQA standards, if improved as recommended, could also be used—by NCQA, the Association for the Accreditation for Human Research Protection Programs (AAHRPP), or other accreditation organizations—as the basis for the development of accreditation standards for non-VA research organizations.

Accreditation will not be successful until it is widely accepted as a mark of excellence. To accomplish this, it should serve as an educational tool to raise the median overall performance of an accredited organization. To do this, accreditation standards and the processes in which they will be used must incorporate consistent feedback from the parties involved in the various aspects of an HRPPP. As discussed above, the local aspects of this issue (i.e., aspects that apply to individual applicant institutions) should be enhanced in the NCQA standards. The committee is encouraged that both NCQA and AAHRPP include stakeholder representatives in their programmatic leaderships (see Recommendation 2). Those who encounter problems in the research protection system, irrespective of the perspective that they represent in that system, need simple, con-

---

[11] Chapter 3 describes some options for research monitoring and feedback. When organizations applying for accreditation conduct research that is monitored by DSMBs, for example, details of how those boards interact with investigators, IRBs, and research administrators would need to be evaluated for all or a representative sample of DSMBs. Reporting mechanisms for severe or unanticipated adverse events would similarly be necessary to evaluate all protocols or a representative sample of protocols. Ombudsman programs and reporting mechanisms for concerns, complaints, and other feedback mechanisms would be included. Pilot testing will likely reveal a wide variety of monitoring and feedback methods that will have to be accommodated in the accreditation process.

[12] PRIM&R's Standard 1.16 calls for assessment of quality improvement programs, and NCQA's standards presented in Table C-3(B) do so with even more specificity. The committee believes that procedures for evaluating the informed-consent process in particular deserve special attention and will be both the foundation of effective protections and the best hope of shifting from documentation to performance measures.

[13] Budget and staffing for IRB operations, monitoring and ombudsman programs, and other HRPPP components are not sufficient to evaluate quality and effectiveness. Insufficient budgets and staffing, however, would be clear indications of deficiencies. The committee sought information about budgets and staffing, but found few data. (The 1998 report by Bell and colleagues contains some data on IRBs and investigators at 491 institutions; it does not, however, include data on IRBs regulated only by the FDA, monitoring bodies, or administrative costs.) Extant data were insufficient for the committee to develop benchmarks for different kinds of organizations seeking accreditation. Such benchmarks will thus have to be established in light of experience from pilot testing.

sistent ways to bring their concerns to light and to bring relevant information into the procedure for the review of the process at the level of both the HRPPP and the accreditation process.

It is the committee's understanding that the NCQA standards will be tested in a pilot study beginning in the spring of 2001.[14] This is an important step in gauging the feasibility of the use of these standards for the accreditation process, and the committee encourages similar pilot testing with appropriately modified standards in non-VA research environments.

---

[14] As this report went to press, NCQA made their draft standards available for public comment. See http://www.ncqa.org/Pages/Programs/QSG/VAHRPAP/vahrpapdraftstds. htm for further information.

4

Evaluating HRPPP Pilot Accreditation Programs

Launching the human research participant protection program (HRPPP) accreditation programs already in motion will take at least a year or two, and it will require at least another year or two of experience before a judgment about the costs and benefits of an accreditation strategy will be possible. Even as the pilot projects are being planned and implemented, however, forethought about how to evaluate them is in order.

Given the nature of the accreditation process, only limited quantitative data are likely to be available at the end of a 3- to 5-year pilot period. Some HRPPPs may have gone out of business. They may choose to contract with a fee-based independent institutional review board (IRB), to affiliate with larger institutions that have operating HRPPPs, or to stop conducting research altogether. The cessation of research because of an inability to demonstrate that research practices respect the rights and interests of research participants is not necessarily an undesirable effect.

The accreditation process will show how many organizations apply for accreditation and what fraction succeed. It is unlikely, however, that the accreditation process itself can produce data that would enable policy makers 5 years from now to make an informed decision about whether accreditation has, on balance, improved the HRPPP system. It is also unlikely that it can produce data on the cost of any enhancement compared with the achievements that could be made by alternative uses of the same resources. The answers to these questions are unlikely to be decided by quantitative data alone, so another evaluation strategy is needed.

Information of two kinds can better guide decisions about improving HRPPPs in general and the role of accreditation in particular. First, a research program is needed both to establish the current baseline (current practices in human research) and to study ways in which that baseline might be improved. Second, the committee believes that an evaluation process that is independent of the Association for the Accreditation of Human Research Protection Programs (AAHRPP), the National Committee for Quality Assurance (NCQA), and any other accreditation bodies that may emerge will be necessary. The committee recommends that federal agencies with a track record of evaluating HRPPPs, such as the U.S. Department of Health and Human Services (DHHS), monitor the accreditation pilot programs.

Recommendation 10: Begin Collecting Data and Assessing Impacts of Accreditation Now

DHHS should commission studies to gather baseline data on the current system of protections for human participants in the re-search that it oversees and to assess whether the system is improv-ing over time.

Baseline data are needed on the following:

• a taxonomy of research institutions: the number of institutions conducting research with human participants and the number of studies of different types (e.g., clinical trials, surveys, student projects, and behavioral studies) approved by their HRPPPs;

• a taxonomy of IRBs: the number of IRBs and what fraction of them are primarily devoted to studies of particular types;

• a taxonomy of studies with humans: the number and distribution of in-vestigations with humans under way by type of study, for example, clinical trials of various stages, observational studies, cross-sectional and longitudinal sur-veys, and social science experiments;

• the number of people involved in research and, among them, how many are involved in research with more than minimal risk;

• the fraction of studies with more than minimal risk that have formal safety monitoring boards and how (and how well) those boards operate;

• the type and number of inquiries, investigations, and sanctions by the Food and Drug Administration and the Office for Human Research Protections; and

• the type and number of serious or unanticipated adverse events attribut-able to research.

DHHS should also commission studies of how the databases for existing clinical trials and other research resources could be used to assess how well the system of research protections is operating and, specifically, whether accreditation is having measurable impacts (e.g., by comparing accredited and nonaccredited institutions or by comparing institutions before and after accreditation).

Other studies are also needed to bolster the nascent literature on how well research participants understand the studies that they join, which risks matter most to them, and what forms of informed consent are most effective. Several new initiatives to enhance clinical research in particular are under way, and the National Institutes of Health has initiated new programs to improve research monitoring. DHHS should evaluate these efforts not only for their primary purpose of improving clinical research but also for how they can improve HRPPPs.

The research pursued under this recommendation should have several uses. It will provide essential data on which to base policy decisions in the future. It will also point to ways in which the system can be improved. It may help assign priorities among strategies to improve the HRPPP system by pointing to strengths and weaknesses in the current system. It is likely to uncover and document problems in the current system, some of which are already known and perhaps others of which are not fully appreciated. Finally, it could reassure the public and policy makers about those aspects of the current system that are functioning well.

Recommendation 11: Initiate Federal Studies Evaluating Accreditation

The U.S. Congress should request an evaluation of accreditation pilot programs from the General Accounting Office. The Secretary of Health and Human Services should consider requesting a parallel evaluation from the Office of the Inspector General of DHHS.

An evaluation process that is independent of AAHRPP, NCQA, and other accreditation bodies can help policy makers decide on the value of accreditation as an improvement strategy several years hence. Without such an evaluation, Congress and the executive branch will be positioned little better than they are today to make prudent choices about how to improve HRPPPs in 5 years. Research pursued under Recommendation 10 can provide some baseline information, but it cannot substitute for a thorough evaluation of the accreditation pilot projects themselves. Furthermore, the evaluation efforts would benefit in several respects if they were initiated soon, while the pilot projects are getting under way. Evaluators could observe which organizations seek accreditation and which ones do not. They could also conduct interviews with organization officials who are making choices to find out why a particular choice was made and what they perceive the benefits or problems of HRPPP accreditation programs to be. If multiple accreditation bodies emerge, the evaluation should compare their effectiveness.

The evaluation methods are likely to be primarily qualitative, supplemented where possible by quantitative data. Interviews, surveys, "shadowing" of IRB staff and accreditation site visit teams, and other methods used while the pilot project is being launched would capture information that is valuable for judging its success or failure and that will otherwise be lost.

The evaluations should take costs of accreditation into account. Accreditation costs in comparable contexts vary over a wide range. The Lewin Group (1998) noted that accreditation for a mammography facility was $900 (plus $1,178 if a site visit was used) whereas accreditation of a hospital by the Joint Commission on Accreditation of Healthcare Organizations was $50,000 (plus $1,500 per inspector per inspection, usually involving three to four inspectors). The 5-year contract between the U.S. Department of Veterans Affairs (VA) and NCQA is $5.8 million (for 141 facilities, or just over $40,000 per facility, 40 of which are affiliated with major research centers), and very preliminary estimates by the nascent AAHRPP anticipated a cost of $15,000 to $20,000 per accreditation cycle (including a site visit to each facility) (David Korn, Association of American Medical Colleges, personal communication, February 2001). These costs are borne by the accredited body. Additional external costs borne by the institutions in preparing for and following up on accreditation are not covered in these estimates, but they may be even higher than direct costs.[1]

The HRPPP accreditation process should be evaluated not only according to whether it has improved protections for human research participants but also according to whether resources devoted to accreditation could be spent to equal or better effect on other ways to improve HRPPP oversight such as education, research monitoring, and improved feedback mechanisms. Evaluation should take into account both the costs of establishing a national accreditation system and the costs to applicant organizations (i.e., both direct and preparatory).

Once complete, evaluations from the General Accounting Office (GAO) or the Office of the Inspector General (OIG) of DHHS, or both, will have to be translated into recommendations for action by the federal government, accreditation bodies, federal and nongovernmental research sponsors, and organizations seeking accreditation. A comparison and synthesis of the findings would be especially important if different evaluations reach slightly different conclusions or make recommendations that differ in detail, which they are likely to do. The

---

[1] The committee sought information about current costs of IRB operations and also about projected costs of accreditation. It judged the best data, such as those in a 1998 report commissioned by NIH (Bell et al., 1998), are too incomplete to form the basis for cost estimates. The AAALAC accreditation program, for example, has eight categories of fees for accreditation and annual maintenance, and a similar fee schedule will likely develop for HRPPPs. In light of the variety of organizations, the incompleteness of cost data, and the fact that the accreditation process outside the VA system has not been specified in any detail, the committee believed it would be premature to specify cost benchmarks now. Such benchmarks should emerge from pilot testing. Estimating overall costs is even more difficult, but will nonetheless have to be part of the evaluation. The value of the accreditation program as a whole will turn on its added value compared to its marginal costs.

National Human Research Protections Advisory Committee (NHRPAC), a new advisory body created with the mission of improving the HRPPP system, has the expertise to perform this task.

Final evaluation reports on the accreditation pilot projects are unlikely before 2005 or 2006, although interim reports may be useful in 2002 or 2003, on the basis of initial experience with the launch phase of the NCQA and AAHRPP accreditation pilot projects (after initial site visits, for example). NHRPAC's charter will expire in June 2002. For NHRPAC to receive and respond to GAO or OIG evaluations with a set of recommendations, its charter would have to be extended. Its authorized staff and funding of one and a half staff members would have to be augmented, at least transiently for 1 year, to perform this function.

Another logical receptor for the OIG and GAO evaluations would be an independent agency to oversee the protection of human participants in research in both the public and the private sectors, if the recommendation of the National Bioethics Advisory Commission to create such an agency is carried out by Congress. In the event that NHRPAC's charter has expired and no independent oversight agency has been formed, then the synthesis of evaluations would have to be carried out by an independent advisory committee created for that purpose or delegated to an existing nongovernmental organization.

References

Accrediting Body for Human Subjects Research Nears Reality. 2001. *Science and Government Report* XXXI(6):1–2.

AAMC (American Association of Medical Colleges). 2000. *Clinical Research: A Reaffirmation of Trust Between Medical Science and the Public.* [Online]. Available http://www.aamc.org/newsroom/pressrel/000608b.htm [accessed February 1, 2001].

AAPP (American Academy of Pharmaceutical Physicians). 2001. Written comments to the Institute of Medicine Committee on Assessing the System for Protecting Human Research Subjects.

AAU (Association of American Universities) Task Force on Research Accountability. 2000. *Report on University Protections of Human Beings Who Are the Subjects of Research.* Washington, DC: AAU. (See also http://www.aau.edu/HumSubRpt06.28.00.pdf).

AAU (Association of American Universities), COGR (Council on Governmental Relations), and NASULGC (National Association of State Universities and Land-Grant Colleges). 2001. Written comments to the Institute of Medicine Committee on Assessing the System for Protecting Human Research Subjects.

AAUP (American Association of University Professors). Forthcoming. *Protecting Human Beings: Institutional Review Boards and Social Science Research.* Draft. Washington, DC: AAUP.

ACHRE (Advisory Committee on Human Radiation Experiments). 1995. *Advisory Committee on Human Radiation Experiments, Final Report.* Washington, DC: U.S. Government Printing Office. (See also http://tis.eh.doe.gov/ohre/roadmap/achre/index.html).

AMA (American Medical Association) Judicial Council. 1946. Supplementary Report of the Judicial Council of the American Medical Association. *Journal of the American Medical Association* 132:1090.

Amdur, R. J. 2000. Improving the Protection of Human Research Subjects. *Academic Medicine* 75:718–720.

Ashe, Warren T. (Associate Dean for Research, Howard University School of Medicine). 2001. Statement at the January 22, 2001, public forum of the Institute of Medicine Committee on Assessing the System for Protecting Human Research Subjects.

Batt, Sharon. 1994. *Patient No More: The Politics of Breast Cancer.* Charlottetown, Prince Edward Island, Canada: Gynergy Books.

Bazell, Robert. 1998. *HER-2: The Making of Herceptin, a Revolutionary Treatment for Breast Cancer.* New York: Random House.

Beecher, Henry K. 1966. Ethics and Clinical Research. *The New England Journal of Medicine* 274:1354–1360.

Bell, James, Whiton, John, and Connelly, Sharon. James Bell Associates. 1998. Prepared for the Office of Extramural Research, NIH. *Evaluation of NIH Implementation of Section 491 of the Public Health Service Act, Mandating a Program of Protection for Research Subjects.* Alexandria, VA: James Bell and Associates.

BNA (Bureau of National Affairs). 1996, December 11. AMA House of Delegate Approves Physician Accreditation Program. *BNA Health Care Daily.* p. d4.

BNA. 2000, April 6. Accreditation Failing to Receive Payer/Provider Support: AMA to Discontinue Accreditation Program. *BNA Health Care Daily.* p. d14.

Case Western Reserve University. 2001. *Office of Research Administration: Human Subjects Protection.* [Online]. Available: http://ora.ra.cwru.edu/main_human_subjects_protection_page.htm [accessed February 15, 2001].

CECHR (Central Ethics Committee on Human Research), Indian Council of Medical Research. 2000. *Ethical Guidelines for Biomedical Research on Human Subjects.* [Online]. Available: http://www.icmr.nic.in/vsicmr/ethical.pdf [accessed January 24, 2001].

Chadwick, Gary, and Liders, Gunta J. 2000. *Re: New Educational Requirements for Human Subject Researchers.* [Online]. Available: http://www.rochester.edu/ORPA/ORPA-L/hsed.html [accessed February 5, 2001].

Chodosh, Sanford (President, Public Responsibility in Medicine and Research). 2000. Statement at the December 18, 2000, meeting of the Institute of Medicine Committee on Assessing the System for Protecting Human Research Subjects.

CIOMS (Council for International Organizations of Medical Sciences). In: Bankowski, Z. and Howard Jones N., eds. 1982. *Human Experimentation and Medical Ethics.* Geneva: CIOMS.

CIOMS. 1993. *International Ethical Guidelines for Biomedical Research Involving Human Subjects.* Geneva: CIOMS.

Clinton, William J. 1995. Protection of Human Research Subjects and Creation of National Bioethics Advisory Commission. Executive Order 12975. *Federal Register* 60(193):52063–52065.

Cook-Deegan, Robert Mullan. 1997. Do Research Moratoria Work? In: *Cloning Human Beings,* Vol. II. *Commissioned Papers.* Rockville, MD: National Bioethics Advisory Commission. Pp. H-1–H-52. (See also www.bioethics.gov/pubs/cloning2/cc8.pdf).

Cornblath, David R (Johns Hopkins Medicine). 2001. Written comments to the Institute of Medicine Committee on Assessing the System for Protecting Human Research Subjects.

DHHS (U.S. Department of Health and Human Services). 2000. *HHS News: New Office for Human Research Protections Created, Dr. Koski Named Director.* [Online]. Available: http://www.hhs.gov/news/press/2000pres/20000606.html [accessed January 15, 2001].

DHHS OIG (U.S. Department of Health and Human Service, Office of Inspector General). 1998a. *Low-Volume Institutional Review Boards.* Publication No. OEI-01-97-00194. (See also http://www.dhhs.gov/progorg/oei/reports/a308.pdf).

DHHS OIG. 1998b. *Institutional Review Boards: A Time for Reform.* Publication No. OEI-01-97-00193. (See also http://www.dhhs.gov/progorg/oei/reports/a276.pdf).

DHHS OIG. 1998c. *Institutional Review Boards: The Emergence of Independent Boards.* Publication No. OEI-01-97-00192. (See also http://www.dhhs.gov/progorg/oei/reports/a275.pdf).

DHHS OIG. 1998d. *Institutional Review Boards: Promising Approaches.* Publication No. OEI-01-97-00191. (See also http://www.dhhs.gov/progorg/oei/reports/a274.pdf).

DHHS OIG. 1998e. *Institutional Review Boards: Their Role in Reviewing Approved Research.* Publication No. OEI-01-97-00190. (See also http://www.dhhs.gov/progorg/oei/reports/a273.pdf).

DHHS OIG. 1999a. *The External Review of Hospital Quality: A Call for Greater Accountability.* Publication No. OEI-01-97-00050. (See also http://www.dhhs.gov/progorg/oei/reports/a381.pdf).

DHHS OIG. 1999b. *The External Review of Hospital Quality: The Role of Accreditation.* Publication No. OEI-01-97-00051. (See also http://www.dhhs.gov/progorg/oei/reports/a382.pdf).

DHHS OIG. 2000a. *FDA Oversight of Clinical Investigators.* Publication No. OEI-05-99-00350. (See also http://www.hhs.gov/oig/oei/reports/a457.pdf).

DHHS OIG. 2000b. *Protecting Human Research Subjects: Status of Recommendations.* Publication No. OEI-01-97-00197. (See also http://www.dhhs.gov/progorg/oei/reports/a447.pdf).

DHHS OIG. 2000c. *Recruiting Human Subjects: Pressures in Industry-Sponsored Clinical Research.* Publication No. OEI-01-97-00195. (See also http://www.hhs.gov/oig/oei/reports/a459.pdf).

DHHS OIG. 2000d. *Recruiting Human Subjects: Sample Guidelines for Practice.* Publication No. OEI-01-97-00196. (See also http://www.hhs.gov/oig/oei/reports/a458.pdf).

Dimmit, Barbara Sande. 1995. Accreditation: What's the Big Deal? *Business and Health* 13:38–44.

Epstein, Steven. 1996. *Impure Science: AIDS, Activism, and the Politics of Knowledge.* Berkeley: University of California Press.

Erickson, Stephen (Director, Office of Research Administration, Boston College). 2001. Statement at the January 22, 2001, hearing of the Institute of Medicine Committee on Assessing the System for Protecting Human Research Subjects.

Faden, Ruth R., and Beauchamp, Tom L. 1986. *A History and Theory of Informed Consent.* New York: Oxford University Press.

Fletcher, John C. Forthcoming. *Location of OPRR Within the NIH: Problems of Status and Independent Authority.* Draft report, the National Bioethics Advisory Commission (NBAC). Rockville, MD: NBAC.

Flexner, Abraham. 1910. *Medical Education in the United States and Canada: A Report to the Carnegie Foundation for the Advancement of Teaching,* Bulletin No. 4. New York: Carnegie Foundation for the Advancement of Teaching.

Gamble, V. N. 1997. Under the Shadow of Tuskegee: African Americans and Health Care. *American Journal of Public Health* 87:1773–1778.

GAO (General Accounting Office). 1996. *Scientific Research: Continued Vigilance Critical to Protecting Human Subjects.* Washington, DC: GAO.

GAO. 2000. *VA Research: Protections for Human Subjects Need to Be Strengthened.* Washington, DC: GAO.

Gelsinger, Paul. 2000. Jesse's Intent. *Guinea Pig Zero* 8:7–17.

Goldschmidt, Peter (President, Medical Care Management Corporation). 2001. Statement at the January 22, 2001, hearing of the Institute of Medicine Committee on Assessing the System for Protecting Human Research Subjects.

Grob, George (Deputy Inspector General for Evaluation and Inspections, Office of Inspector General, U. S. Department of Health and Human Services). 2000. *Testimony on Protecting Human Subjects: Status of Recommendations.* Statement at the May 3, 2000, hearing of the Subcommittee on Criminal Justice, Drug Policy and Human Resources, Committee on Government Reform, U.S. House of Representatives. (See also http://www.house.gov/reform/cj/hearings/00.05.03/Grob.htm).

Gunsalus, C. K. Forthcoming. *An Examination of Issues Presented by Proposal to Unify and Expand Federal Oversight of Human Subject Research.* Draft report for the National Bioethics Advisory Commission (NBAC). Rockville, MD: NBAC.

Hamm, Michael. 1997. *The Fundamentals of Accreditation.* Washington, DC: American Society of Association Executives.

Hanna, K. E. 2000. Research Ethics: Reports, Scandals, Calls for Change. *The Hastings Center Report* 30(6):6.

Heller, J. 1972. Syphilis Victims in U.S. Study Went Untreated for 40 Years. *The New York Times.* p. A1.

International Conference on Harmonisation of Technical Requirements for Registration of Pharmaceuticals for Human Use. 1996. *Therapeutic Products Directorate Guidelines: ICH Harmonised Tripartite Guideline: General Considerations for Clinical Trials.* Ottawa, Canada: Health Canada. (See also http://www.hc-sc.gc.ca/hpb-dgps/therapeut/zfiles/english/guides/ich/efficacy/gclintr_e.html)

International Conference on Harmonisation of Technical Requirements for Registration of Pharmaceuticals for Human Use. 1997. *Therapeutic Products Directorate Guidelines: ICH Harmonised Tripartite Guideline: Good Clinical Practice: Consolidated Guideline.* Ottawa, Canada: Health Canada. (See also http://www.hc-sc.gc.ca/hpb-dgps/therapeut/zfiles/english/guides/ich/efficacy/goodclin_e.html)

International Conference on Harmonisation. 1998. *International Conference on Harmonisation Structure.* [Online]. Available: http://www.ifpma.org/ich2.html [accessed February 22, 2001].

IOM (Institute of Medicine). 1994. In: Mastroianni, Anna C., Faden, Ruth, and Federman, Daniel, ed. *Women and Health Research: Ethical and Legal Issues of Including Women in Clinical Studies.* Washington, DC: National Academy Press.

IOM. 1999. *The Unequal Burden of Cancer: An Assessment of NIH Research and Programs for Ethnic Minorities and the Medically Underserved.* Washington, DC: National Academy Press.

IOM. 2001. Public forum of the Institute of Medicine Committee on Assessing the System for Protecting Human Research Subjects. January 22, 2001.

Isidor, John (CEO, Shulman and Associates IRB, Inc.). 2001. Statement at the January 22, 2001, hearing of the Institute of Medicine Committee on Assessing the System for Protecting Human Research Subjects.

JCAHO (Joint Commission on Accreditation of Healthcare Organizations). 2000. *Joint Commission Standards*. [Online]. Available: www.jcaho.org/standard/jcstandards. html [accessed February 13, 2001].

Jones, J. H. 1981. *Bad Blood: The Tuskegee Syphilis Experiment*. New York: The Free Press.

Jost, Timothy. 1994. Medicare and the Joint Commission on Accreditation of Healthcare Organizations: A Healthy Relationship? *Law and Contemporary Problems* 57:15–46.

Kant, Immanuel. 1999. The Good Will. In: Feinberg, J., and Shafer-Landau, R., ed. *Reason and Responsibility*. Belmont, CA: Wadsworth Publishing Company. pp. 558–570.

Kulakowski, Elliott C. (President, Society of Research Administrators International). 2001. Written comments to the Institute of Medicine Committee on Assessing the System for Protecting Human Research Subjects.

Lehrman, Sally. 2000a. The Gelsinger Story. [Online]. *GeneLetter*. Available: http://www.geneletter.com/05-01-00/features/gelsinger1.html [accessed February 20, 2001].

Lehrman, Sally. 2000b. The Gelsinger Story: Aftermath. [Online]. *GeneLetter*. Available: http://www.geneletter.com/06-01-00/features/gelsinger2.html [accessed February 20, 2001].

Levine, Felice J. (American Sociological Association and Consortium of Social Science Associations). 2001. Statement at the January 22, 2001, hearing of the Institute of Medicine Committee on Assessing the System for Protecting Human Research Subjects.

Lewin Group. Prepared for the Center for Substance Abuse Treatment. 1998. *Profiling Regulatory Models*. Fairfax, Virginia: The Lewin Group, Inc.

Love, Susan M. 1995. *Dr. Susan Love's Breast Book*. 2nd ed. Reading, MA: Perseus Books.

Marshall, Patricia A. Forthcoming. *The Relevance of Culture for Informed Consent in U.S. Funded International Health Research*. Draft Report for the National Bioethics Advisory Commission (NBAC). Rockville, MD: NBAC.

Mastroianni, Anna C., and Kahn, Jeffrey P. 1998. The Importance of Expanding Current Training in the Responsible Conduct of Research. *Academic Medicine* 73:1249–1254.

McCarthy, Charles R. Forthcoming. *Reflections on the Organizational Locus of the Office for Protection from Research Risks*. Draft Report for the National Bioethics Advisory Commission (NBAC). Rockville, MD: NBAC.

Merkatz, Ruth B., and Summers, Elyse I. 1997. Including Women in Clinical Trials: Policy Changes at the Food and Drug Administration. In: Haseltine, Florence P., Greenberg Jacobson, Beverly, and Society for the Advancement of Women's Health Research, ed. *Women's Health Research: A Medical and Policy Primer*. Washington, DC: Health Press International.

National Association of IRB Managers. 2001. *About the Program*. [Online]. Available: www.naim.org/cert.htm [accessed March 27, 2001].

National Commission for the Protection of Human Subjects of Biomedical and Behavioral Research. 1979. *The Belmont Report: Ethical Principles and Guidelines for the Protection of Human Subjects of Research*. Washington, DC: U.S. Government Printing Office.

NBAC (National Bioethics Advisory Commission). 1997. *Cloning Human Beings*, Volume I. Rockville, MD: U.S. Government Printing Office. (See also http://bioethics. gov/pubs/cloning1/cloning.pdf).

NBAC. 1998. *Research Involving Persons with Mental Disorders That May Affect Decisionmaking Capacity.* Rockville, MD: U.S. Government Printing Office. (See also http://bioethics.gov/capacity/TOC.htm).

NBAC. 1999a. *Research Involving Human Biological Materials: Ethical Issues and Policy Guidance.* Rockville, MD: U.S. Government Printing Office. (See also http://bioethics.gov/hbm.pdf).

NBAC. 1999b. *Ethical Issues in Human Stem Cell Research.* Rockville, MD: U.S. Government Printing Office. (See also http://bioethics.gov/stemcell.pdf).

NBAC. Forthcoming-a. *Ethical and Policy Issues in International Research.* Draft. Rockville, MD: U.S. Government Printing Office. (See also http://bioethics.gov/ toc_pdf).

NBAC. Forthcoming-b. *Ethical and Policy Issues in Research Involving Human Participants.* Draft. (See also http://bioethics.gov/human/human_comment.html).

NCI (National Cancer Institute). 1997. *Report of the National Cancer Institute Clinical Trials Program Review Group (The Armitage Report).* [Online]. Available: http://deainfo.nci.nih.gov/advisory/bsa/bsa_program/2a [accessed February 5, 2001].

NCI. 1999. Monitoring of Clinical Trials. [Online]. *NIH Guide for Grants and Contracts: Notices.* Available: http://grants.nih.gov/grants/guide/notice-files/not99-140.html [accessed February 5, 2001].

NCI. 2001. *Cancer Clinical Trials: A New National System.* [Online]. Available: http:// cancertrials.nci.nih.gov/system/html/newsystem.html [accessed February 5, 2001].

NCQA (National Committee for Quality Assurance). 2001a. *MCO Accreditation Information.* [Online]. Available: http://www.ncqa.org/Pages/Programs/Accreditation/ mco/accred.htm [accessed February 1, 2001].

NCQA. 2001b. *VA Human Research Accreditation Program.* [Online]. Available: http:// www.ncqa.org/Pages/Programs/QSG/vahrpap.htm [accessed January 11, 2001].

NIH (National Institutes of Health). 2000. *Further Guidance on a Data and Safety Monitoring for Phase I and Phase II Trials.* [Online]. Available: http://grants.nih. gov/grants/guide/notice-files/NOT-OD-00-038.html [accessed February 2, 2001].

Nishimi, Robyn Y. (Senior Associate, Office of Technology Assessment). 1994. Statement at the September 28, 1994, hearing of the Subcommittee on Legislation and National Security, Committee on Government Operations, U.S. House of Representatives.

NRC (National Research Council). 1996. *Guide for the Care and Use of Laboratory Animals.* Washington, DC: National Academy Press.

NSERC (Natural Sciences and Engineering Research Council of Canada). 2000. *NSERC-Tri-Council Policy Statement: Ethical Conduct of Research Involving Humans.* [Online]. Available: http://www.nserc.ca/programs/ethics/english. [accessed February 22, 2001].

Nuremberg Code. 1949. In: *Trials of War Criminals Before the Nuremberg Military Tribunals Under Control Council Law No. 10.* Nuremberg, October 1946–April 1949. Washington, DC: U.S. Government Printing Office.

Oakes, David D. (Chair, Administrative Panel on Human Subjects in Medical Research, Stanford University), 2001. Written comments to the Institute of Medicine Committee on Assessing the System for Protecting Human Research Subjects.

Office for Protection from Research Risks Review Panel. 1999. *Report to the Advisory Committee to the Director, NIH from the Office for Protection from Research Risks Review Panel.* Rockville, MD: National Institutes of Health. (See also http://www.nih.gov/about/director/060399b.htm.)

Office of Human Subjects Research, National Institutes of Health. 2001. *Protection of Human Research Subjects Computer-Based Training for Researchers.* [Online]. Available: http://ohsr.od.nih.gov/cbt [accessed February 5, 2001].

OHRP. 2000a. *Registration of an Institutional Review Board (IRB) or Independent Ethics Committee (IEC): C.2.* [Online]. Available: http://ohrp.osophs.dhhs.gov/humansubjects/assurance/INTL [accessed February 22, 2001].

OHRP. 2000b. *Procedures for Registering Institutional Review Boards (IRBs) and Filing Federalwide Assurances of Protection for Human Subjects.* [Online]. Available: http://ohrp.osophs.dhhs.gov/irbasur.htm [accessed January 31, 2001].

OMB (Office of Management and Budget). 1998. *Circular No. A-119, Revised.* [Online]. Available: www.whitehouse.gov/omb/circulars/a119/a119.html [accessed February 28, 2001].

OTA (Office of Technology Assessment), U.S. Congress. 1993. *Biomedical Ethics in U.S. Public Policy—Background Paper.* Washington, DC: U.S. Government Printing Office. (See also http://www.wws.princeton.edu/cgi-bin/byteserv.prl/~ota/disk1/1993/9312/9312.pdf.)

Overbey, Mary Margaret (Director of Government Relations, American Anthropological Association). 2001. Written comments to the Institute of Medicine Committee on Assessing the System for Protecting Human Research Subjects.

PHS (U.S. Public Health Service). 1966. Clinical Investigations Using Human Subjects. In: *Final Report: Advisory Committee on Human Radiation Experiments, Supplemental Volume I.* Washington, DC: U.S. Government Printing Office. Pp. 475–476.

President's Commission (President's Commission for the Study of Ethical Problems in Medicine and Biomedical and Behavioral Research). 1981. *Protecting Human Subjects: The Adequacy and Uniformity of Federal Rules and Their Implementation.* Washington, DC: U.S. Government Printing Office.

President's Commission. 1983. *Implementing Human Research Regulations: The Adequacy and Uniformity of Federal Rules and of Their Implementation.* Washington, DC: U.S. Government Printing Office.

PRIM&R (Public Responsibility in Medicine and Research). 2001a. *IRB Professional Certification Exam.* [Online]. Available: http://www.primr.org/certification.html [accessed February 13, 2001].

PRIM&R. 2001b. *AAAHRP Update.* [Online]. Available: http://www.primr.org/aahrppupdate.html [accessed February 19, 2001].

Rettig, Richard A. 2000. The Industrialization of Clinical Research. *Health Affairs* 19:129–146.

Rothman, David J. 1991. *Strangers at the Bedside: A History of How Law and Bioethics Transformed Medical Decision Making.* New York: Basic Books.

Rubin, Philip (Director, Division of Behavioral and Cognitive Sciences, National Science Foundation). 2001. Statement at the January 22, 2001, hearing of the Institute of Medicine Committee on Assessing the System for Protecting Human Research Subjects.

Rudder, Catherine (Executive Director, American Political Science Association). 2001. Written comments to the Institute of Medicine Committee on Assessing the System for Protecting Human Research Subjects.

Ryan, Stephen J. (Dean, Keck School of Medicine, University of Southern California). 2001. Written comments to the Institute of Medicine Committee on Assessing the System for Protecting Human Research Subjects.

Shalala, Donna. 2000. Sounding Board: Protecting Research Subjects—What Must Be Done. *New England Journal of Medicine* 343: 808–810.

Shopes, Linda (Historian, Pennsylvania Historical and Museum Commission). 2001. Written comments to the Institute of Medicine Committee on Assessing the System for Protecting Human Research Subjects.

Snyderman, R., and Holmes E. W. 2000. Oversight Mechanisms for Clinical Research. *Science* 287:595–597.

Starr, Paul. 1982. *Transformation of American Medicine: The Rise of a Sovereign Profession and the Making of a Vast Industry.* New York: Basic Books.

Sugarman, J. 2000. The Role of Institutional Support in Protecting Human Research Subjects. *Academic Medicine* 75:687–692.

Thompson, Larry. 1994. *Correcting the Code: Inventing the Genetic Cure for the Human Body.* New York: Simon and Schuster.

Tuskegee Syphilis Study Ad Hoc Advisory Panel. 1973. *Final Report.* Washington, DC: U.S. Department of Health, Education, and Welfare.

United States v. *Karl Brandt* et al. 1949. In: *The Medical Case, Trials of War Criminals Before the Nuremberg Military Tribunals Under Control Council Law No. 10.* Washington, DC: U.S. Government Printing Office.

U.S. House of Representatives, Committee on Veterans Affairs. 1999. *Suspension of Medical Research at West Los Angeles and Sepulveda VA Medical Facilities and Informed Consent and Patient Safety in VA Medical Research: Hearing of the Committee on Veterans Affairs.* 106th Cong. April 21, 1999.

U.S. Senate, Subcommittee on Public Health, Committee on Health, Education, Labor, and Pensions. 2000. *Gene Therapy: Is There Oversight for Patient Safety?: Hearing of the Subcommittee on Public Health, Committee on Health, Education, Labor, and Pensions.* 106th Congress. February 2, 2000.

VA (U.S. Department of Veterans Affairs). 2000. *Press Release: VA Raises Standard for Protecting Human Research Participants.* [Online]. Available: http://www.va.gov/opa [accessed February 20, 2001].

Weiss, R. and Nelson, D. 1999, December 8. Methods Faulted in Fatal Gene Therapy. *The Washington Post.* p. A1.

World Medical Association. 1964. *Declaration of Helsinki: Ethical Principles for Medical Research Involving Human Subjects.* Ferney-Voltaire, France: World Medical Association.

World Medical Association. 2000. *Declaration of Helsinki: Ethical Principles for Medical Research Involving Human Subjects, revised.* Ferney-Voltaire, France: World Medical Association.

Young, Kenneth E., Chamber, Charles M., Kells, H. R., and Associates. 1983. *Understanding Accreditation.* San Francisco: Jossey-Bank, Inc.

Appendixes

APPENDIX A

Data Sources and Methods

In an effort to comprehensively address the task of recommending accreditation standards for Human Research Participant Protection Programs (HRPPPs), the committee reviewed and considered various data sources in a concerted effort to cast a broad net for the collection and assessment of information. These sources included presentations before the committee from interested organizations, individuals, and federal agencies as well as formal public comments; a review of relevant literature; and commissioned draft standards for accreditation. A summary description of the committee's evidence-gathering methods follows.

PRESENTATIONS AND PUBLIC COMMENT

Over the course of the study, the committee requested and received written responses and presentations from organizations and individuals representing many perspectives of accreditation and human subjects protections in general. The committee felt it was important to receive as much input as possible from public and private groups involved with or seeking involvement in the accreditation process and human subjects protections, as well as from health professional and other organizations. To accomplish this, the committee held public meetings on December 18, 2000, and February 21, 2001, and convened a larger public forum on January 22, 2001, to gather information and hear from groups and individuals. The speakers at these meetings are listed in Box A-1.

BOX A-1 Organizations and Individuals Appearing Before the Committee

December 18, 2000
Sanford Chodosh, Public Responsibility in Medicine and Research
Michael Hamm, Michael Hamm and Associates
David Korn, Association of American Medical Colleges
Greg Koski, HHS Office for Human Research Protections
Charles McCarthy, Kennedy Institute of Ethics
Richard Rettig, RAND Corporation
Marjorie Speers, National Bioethics Advisory Commission
Mark Yessian, HHS Office of Inspector General

January 22, 2001
Jessica Briefer French, National Committee for Quality Assurance
Jim Burris, Department of Veterans Affairs
Marie M. Cassidy, Citizens for Responsible Care and Research
Steve Erickson, Boston College
William L. Freeman, Indian Health Service
Edward F. Gabriele, Naval Medical Research Center
Peter Goldschmidt, Medical Care Management Corporation
Vera Hassner Sharav, Citizens for Responsible Care and Research
John Isidor, Shulman and Associates IRB, Inc.
Jonathan Knight, American Association of University Professors
David Lepay, Food and Drug Administration
Felice Levine, American Sociological Association/Consortium of Social
    Science Associations
John R. Livengood, Centers for Disease Control and Prevention
Barbara J. LoDico, University of Medicine and Dentistry of New Jersey
Dan Masys, University of California, San Diego
Cherlyn Mathias, Private citizen
Nick Reuter, Substance Abuse and Mental Health Services Administration
Philip Rubin, National Science Foundation
John Smith, Morehouse School of Medicine
David P. Stevens, Association of American Medical Colleges
Irene Stith-Coleman, Department of Health and Human Services
Margaret VanAmringe, Joint Commission on Accreditation of Health
    Organizations
Myrl Weinberg, National Health Council

February 21, 2001
Greg Koski, HHS Office for Human Research Protections
Belinda Seto, NIH Office of Extramural Research

During the first committee meeting, a number of speakers addressed the history of human subjects protections and the industrialization of clinical research and provided overviews of the HHS Office of Inspector General activities, the HHS Office of Human Research Protections (OHRP), and accreditation processes among other topics.

At the second meeting, the committee convened a public forum in order to hear a variety of perspectives on the preliminary draft accreditation standards formulated by Public Responsibility in Medicine and Research (PRIM&R), the accreditation process, and the protection of human research subjects. Over 125 people attended the meeting. Representatives of government and regulatory organizations, private accrediting groups, associations, institutions, IRBs, social science groups, research participants, and investigators made short presentations that were subject to comment and questioning from the committee and audience.

In order to include as many people and groups as possible, the committee sent out a mailing that included an announcement of the public forum, a one-page description of the study, the committee roster, and a cover letter explaining the committee's purpose for requesting the information. The letter was sent to a variety of interested people and groups via fax, e-mail, and listservs, and asked those interested to send or fax comments pertinent to the committee's task and to respond to the PRIM&R draft standards for accreditation. The committee also used the project website [www.iom.edu/hrrp] to elicit comments on the project and the draft standards by providing project details, contacts, and links to pertinent information. The materials submitted to the committee supplemented those obtained by the committee through the literature review and public meetings.

A small portion of the third committee meeting was held in open session to hear additional comments from project sponsors.

In addition to the participants listed in Box A-1, many other individuals attended and participated in the public meetings, and/or provided written information to the committee. All registered participants for the January 2001 forum are listed below:

Aronson, Debra
Private citizen

Ashe, Warren K.
Howard University School of
  Medicine

Bailey, Veronica
Children's Hospital,
Washington, D.C. IRB

Berger, Douglas
National Bioethics Advisory
Commission

Brooks, Tricia
Capitol Associates, Inc.

Brown, Rachel
Association of Independent
  Research Institutes

Bruinooge, Suanna S.
American Society of Clinical
  Oncology

Burkom, Diane
Battelle Centers for Public Health
  Research and Evaluation

Byerly, Wesley G.
Wake Forest University School of
  Medicine

Caia, Matt
Committee on National Statistics,
National Academy of Sciences

Cantor, Michael
Veterans Health Administration
National Center for Ethics

Carley, John M.
U.S. Environmental Protection
    Agency

Carpentier, Richard
National Council on Ethics in
    Human Research

Chesley, Francis D., Jr.
Agency for Healthcare Research
    and Quality

Chodosh, Sanford
Public Responsibility in
    Medicine and Research

Cohen, Jeffrey
Office for Human Research
    Protections

Coleman, Laura
Eli Lilly and Co.

Cuccherini, Brenda A.
Veterans Health Administration

Daly, Nancy
American Society of Therapeutic
    Radiology and Oncology

DeCrappeo, Anthony
Council on Governmental
    Relations

DeRenzo, Evan G
Washington Hospital Center

Dessaint, Danelle
Division of Behavioral and Social
    Sciences and Education, NAS

deWolf, Virginia A.
NRC Committee on National
    Statistics

Dinsdale, Henry
National Council on Ethics in
    Human Research

Dong, Bertha
U.S. General Accounting Office

Dunn, Cindy M.
University of Rochester

Dustira, Alicia K.
Office of Research Integrity

Eaglen, Robert
Liaison Committee on Medical
    Education

Eckenwiler, Lisa A.
Old Dominion University

Erickson, Stephen
Boston College

Feldman, Laura S.
National Association of Children's
    Hospitals

Fish, Bob
U.S. Army Medical Research and
    Materiel Command

Fleming, Yolanda A.
National Medical Association

Foote, Donna
Newsweek Magazine

Furtek, Edward
University of California, San Diego

Gallegos, Alice
SUNY Stony Brook

Gasparis, George
Office of Human Research
    Protections

Gelb, Romy
U.S. General Accounting Office

Gemski, Liz
Capitol Associates

Goebel, Paul W., Jr.
Office of Human Research
    Protections

Gordon, Daniel M.
Walter Reed Army Institute of
    Research

Gordon, Valery M.
Office of Extramural Programs,
    OER, OD, NIH

Gottfried, Kate
Office for Human Research Pro-
    tections

Graziano, Alfred S., Jr.
U.S. Air Force

Gross, Lauren G.
American Association of
    Immunologists

Hamm, Michael
Michael Hamm and
    Associates/PRIM&R

Han, Sang
National Association of State
    Universities and Land-Grant
    Colleges

Harpel, Richard
National Association of State
    Universities and Land-Grant
    Colleges

Hartnett, Terry
Clinical Trials Advisor

Hauck, Robert J. P.
American Political Science
    Association

Higgins, Yvonne K.
U.S. Air Force

Hurt, Valerie
Private citizen

Kalf, George F.
Thomas Jefferson University

Kaneshiro, Julie
Office of Science Policy, NIH

Kester, Kent E.
Walter Reed Institute of Research

Khin-Maung-Gyi, Felix
Chesapeake Research Review, Inc.

Kohn, Adam M.
Shaw Pittman

Kuehl, Patricia
PAREXEL International

Kulakowski, Elliott C.
Society of Research Administrators
  International/
Albert Einstein Healthcare
  Network

Lechter, Karen
Food and Drug Administration

Lee, Bonnie M.
Food and Drug Administration

Levine, Jen
Washington Drug Letter

Linde-Serge, Marian
Food and Drug Administration

Lorden, Joan F.
University of Alabama at
  Birmingham

Macko, Gail
Tactical Research, LLC

McFarland, Jeff
Society of Research Administrators
  International

Meyer, Roger E.
Association of American Medical
  Colleges

Milstein, Alan
Sherman, Silverstein, Kohl, Rose &
  Podolsky

Mitchell, Marcus
Glaxo-SmithKline

Mitchell, Mary H.
Harvard University

Morgan, Charlene
Department of the Navy, Bureau of
  Medicine and Surgery

Nightingale, Stuart
Department of Health and Human
  Services

Noble, Gary R.
Johnson & Johnson

Noble, John H., Jr.
Catholic University of America

Okie, Susan
Washington Post

Overbey, Mary Margaret
American Anthropological
  Association

Panicker, Sangeeta
American Psychological
  Association

Papagni, Paul
Columbia University/New York
  Presbyterian Medical Center

Patel, Nilam
Agency for Healthcare Research
  and Quality

Patterson, Wayne
The University of Texas Medical
  Branch at Galveston

Paulsen, Cindy
University of Chicago

Perricord, Douglas
Quintiles Transnational

Polmar, Suzanne K.
Yale University

Pospisil, George C.
National Institute of Neurological
  Disorders and Stroke, NIH

Powell, James H.
National Medical Association

Puglisi, Tom
PricewaterhouseCoopers

Radcliffe, Sara
PhRMA

Reid, Ken
Bioresearch Monitoring Report

Russel-Einhorn, Michele
PricewaterhouseCoopers

Sanford, Sandra
NCQA

Scanley, Anne
National Institute of Allergy and
  Infectious Diseases

Scharke, Cliff
Office for Human Research
  Protections

Schrode, Kristi
Bennet, Turner & Coleman, LLP

Schwartz, Harvey A.
Agency for Healthcare Research
  and Quality

Seto, Belinda
National Institutes of Health

Shamoo, Adil E.
University of Maryland School of
  Medicine

Sharpe, Angela
Consortium of Social Science
  Associations

Shawver, Mary N.
Diamond Healthcare Corporation

Sherwin, Joseph R.
University of Pennsylvania

Siang, Sanyin
American Association for the
  Advancement of Science

Silver, Howard J.
Consortium of Social Science
  Associations

Simonson, Kristin
American Society of Therapeutic
  Radiology and Oncology

Skedvold, Paula
National Institutes of Health
Office of Behavioral and Social
  Sciences Research

Skelton, Margaret Ann
School of Medicine and Health
  Sciences,
George Washington University

Smedberg, Paul
National Health Council

Spilker, Bert
PhRMA

Stith-Coleman, Irene
Department of Health and Human
  Services

Straf, Miron L.
Directorate for Social, Behavioral,
  and Economic Sciences,
National Science Foundation

Studer, Evelyn
Research Triangle Institute

Swanson, Dennis
University of Pittsburgh
Institutional Review Board

Turman, Richard J.
Association of American
  Universities

Vincent, Angela
National Medical Association

Waterman, Paula
Department of Veterans Affairs,
  Office of Research Compliance
  and Assurance

Weiner, Susan L.
The Children's Cause, Inc.

Wenner, Karen A.
McKesson HBOC Pharmaceutical
  Partners Group

Wichman, Alison
NIH Office of Human Subjects
  Research

Wingard, Jennifer
National Association of State Universities and Land Grant Colleges

Zarin, Deborah
Agency for Healthcare Research
  and Quality

Zimmerman, Janet F.
IMPACT Consulting Group

The following people and organizations submitted written comments to the committee about accreditation programs and/or the PRIM&R Standards:

American Political Science
  Association

Association of American Universi-
  ties/Council on Governmental
  Relations/National Association
  of State Universities and Land
  Grant Colleges

Citizens for Responsible
Care & Research

Cornblath, David R.
Johns Hopkins Medicine

Eckenwiler, Lisa A.
Old Dominion University

Erickson, Stephen
Boston College

Feussner, John R.
Department of Veterans Affairs,
Veterans Health Administration

Freeman, William
Indian Health Service

Gabriele, Edward F.
Naval Medical Research Center

Kulakowski, Elliott C.
Society of Research Administrators
International

Levine, Felice J.
American Sociological Associa-
tion/Consortium of Social
Science Associations

National Medical Association

Oakes, David D.
Stanford University

Overbey, Mary Margaret
American Anthropological
Association

Patterson, Wayne
The University of Texas Medical
Branch at Galveston

Richards, R. Henry
American Academy of
Pharmaceutical Physicians

Rubin, Phillip
National Science Foundation

Ryan, Stephen J.
University of Southern California

Swanson, Dennis
University of Pittsburgh

Shopes, Linda
Pennsylvania Historical & Museum
Commission

Townsend, Ardis Noreen
Private citizen

Vasgird, Daniel R.
Research Foundation of the City
University of New York

Weinberg, Myrl
National Health Council

All written materials presented to the committee were reviewed and considered with respect to the task. This material can be examined by the public. The public access files are maintained by the National Research Council Library at 2001 Wisconsin Avenue, N.W., Harris Building, Room HA 152, Washington, DC 20007; tel: (202) 334-3543.

LITERATURE REVIEW

In order to be thorough in their review, the committee conducted multiple literature searches and read numerous articles, book chapters, and reports concerning the protection of human subjects of research and its components during the course of the study. The materials provided addressed topics including the history of human subjects protections; the laws, processes, and groups that regulate human research; critiques of the current system for protecting human research subjects; sample accreditation programs; and ethical issues surrounding human research.

DRAFT STANDARDS FOR ACCREDITATION

Due to the fast-track nature of this study, the Institute of Medicine sought to assist the committee in completing its task in a timely manner. For this reason, the IOM funded the completion of a two-year effort by PRIM&R to establish accreditation standards. The resulting standards were intended to assist the committee in its deliberations about accreditation strategies and their strengths and weaknesses.

In addition, in the course of the committee's analysis, the draft standards developed by NCQA under contract with the Department of Veterans Affairs were provided to the committee for inclusion in their assessment of accreditation standards.

APPENDIX B

PRIM&R Accreditation Standards

INTRODUCTION

The research community, Congress, and the public have all voiced concerns regarding the adequacy of the system for the protection of human research participants. In response to these concerns, and to suspensions of research at a few institutions around the country, in May 1999 Public Responsibility in Medicine and Research (PRIM&R) began the development of a proposed accreditation program. The accreditation program would be voluntary and educationally driven, directed toward improving human subject protection programs and thereby promoting the strongest possible system of protections for individuals studied in research.

The planned accreditation program has two phases: The first phase has been the development and planned promulgation of objective, outcome-oriented performance standards, which can then serve as the measurement criteria for the new private, voluntary accreditation program described above. Beginning in the fall of 1999, PRIM&R convened a multi-disciplinary group of individuals, all of whom have been leaders in their respective fields, to write these draft Standards. Four writing group "retreats" were held, and the balance of the work was conducted via telephone and e-mail.

Once these standards have been reviewed and accepted, they will be suitable for both self-assessment and formal peer review during the accreditation process. With respect to their self-assessment function, it is expected that the standards will serve as a guidepost to aid organizations and other entities in building and/or strengthening their programs for the protection of protections for individuals studied in research.

The on-site review portion of the accreditation program is the second phase, and, as mentioned above, be voluntary, educational, and constructive.

Standards are prerequisite to the successful operation of an accreditation system, as they provide a means by which expectations can be stated, and by which performance in accordance with those expectations can be measured.

When evaluating the applicability of these standards to a given research program, the responsible institutional individual(s) should take into account the types of research with which that human research protection program is involved. For example, in light of the continuing increase of multicenter and cooperative studies, organizations participating in such trials must first assess the manner in which the various components of their Human Research Protection Program interact in order to provide appropriate protective mechanisms.

GOALS

The goal of voluntary accreditation is to improve the systems that protect the rights and safeguard the welfare of individuals who participate in research. Secondary goals may include:

• To communicate to the scientific community and to the public a strong declaration of a research organization's commitment to the protection of human research participants;

• To help organizations understand the need to commit adequate resources to maintain quality human research protection programs;

• To enhance an organization's ability to attract students to graduate research training programs; and

• To promote a higher quality of research, which will in turn result in better scientific outcomes and, ultimately, better healthcare.

PRINCIPLES UNDERLYING THE PROTECTION OF
HUMANS STUDIED IN RESEARCH

In the United States the conduct of research involving humans is a conditional privilege requiring that research is conducted in keeping with well-established ethical principles, applicable federal, state, and local laws, and/or relevant policies and procedures.

The Belmont Report—Ethical Principles and Guidelines for the Protection of Human Subjects of Research (1979) provides the philosophical basis for current laws governing human subjects research. This Report identifies three fundamental ethical principles that are relevant to all research involving human subjects: (1) Respect for Persons, (2) Beneficence, and (3) Justice. Application of these principles in the conduct of human research requires: (1) that the process of informed consent be prerequisite to an individual's participation; (2) that additional protections be employed for persons who cannot provide this consent; (3) that risks and benefits be responsibly and ethically assessed; (4) that research populations have been selected equitably; and (5) that equity exists for all individuals in consideration of the burdens and benefits of the research. Each of these principles carries equal moral force, and difficult ethical dilemmas may arise when they conflict.

Careful and thoughtful application of the principles of *The Belmont Report* cannot be exclusively relied upon to resolve particular ethical problems without conflict. The principles, however, do provide an analytical framework that will help guide the resolution of most ethical problems arising during the development and review of research, and that will increase the likelihood that individuals who agree to be studied in research will be treated in an ethical manner.

These voluntary accreditation standards incorporate the ethical principles of *The Belmont Report*. Therefore, seeking accreditation is an organization's public declaration that it endorses and implements the Belmont principles.

GLOSSARY

Accreditation An assessment process in which an agency uses experts in a particular field of interest or discipline to define standards of acceptable and applicable operation/performance for an organization/system and to measure compliance with them.

Data and Safety Monitoring Board (DSMB) A group of experts, independent of the research project, who review the safety data and critical efficacy endpoints of a research protocol at specified intervals and recommend whether to continue, modify, or terminate that research. It should be noted that DSMBs are usually convened in phase III and in large multicenter studies, and not routinely in phase I and II trials. In addition, it should be noted that a DSMB should not be confused with a data and safety monitoring plan, which is required for all NIH clinical trials.

Human Research Protection Program (HRPP) A system that includes all components critical to protecting individuals studied in research and that is managed in accordance with these standards and with applicable federal, state, and local laws and regulations. In general, the HRPP has a central authority, Institutional Review Board(s) (IRB), IRB staff, and researchers and research personnel. Some components of the HRPP may be external to the organization seeking accreditation, but the essential components of an HRPP should be identifiable in all cases.

Institutional/Organizational Official An individual within the organization who has the responsibility for and authority over the Human Research Protection Program (HRPP).

Institutional Review Boards (IRBs) Committees or boards that review research to ensure the protection of human subjects. The term includes, but is not limited to Institutional Review Boards (per the Common Rule, 45 CFR 46), Central Review Boards, Independent Review Boards, and Cooperative Research Boards.

Investigator Any individual who has responsibility for the design, conduct, management, or analysis of research.

Organization The entity with an HRPP. Organizations include but are not limited to corporations, private research entities, hospitals, universities, colleges, institutions, and governmental agencies. The functional arrangement of the HRPP may vary depending upon the type of organization. There are circumstances when the sponsor of the research (e.g., a pharmaceutical firm) may be the logical organization responsible for the HRPP.

Research A systematic investigation, including research development, testing, and evaluation, designed to develop or contribute to generalizable knowledge, or, any experiment that involves an FDA-regulated test article.

Research Participant/Subject/Individual Studied in Research An individual about whom an investigator conducting research obtains (1) data through intervention or interaction with the individual, or (2) identifiable private information. The term "subject" is traditionally used in the literature and in federal regulations to describe these individuals. In these Standards, the term "subject" will be used when the individual has not had an opportunity to consent to the research, "participant" or "research participant" will be used when the individual has consented to be part of the research, and "individual studied in research" will be used in a general sense when either may be the case.

Sponsor Any entity that provides funds or other resources to support the research. This entity could be a federal agency, corporation, foundation, institution, or an individual.

PROPOSED STANDARDS

Section 1—Organizational Responsibilities

1.1 Protection of individuals studied in research must be a core value within the organization.

COMMENTARY on Standard 1.1: Officials at the highest level of the governing body of an organization shall demonstrate to the organization the importance and value of the protection of the individuals studied in research by the development and support of a system of protections. This principle should become a basic tenet in the organization.

1.2   The organization must uphold ethical principles underlying the protection of individuals studied in research.
COMMENTARY on Standard 1.2: *The Belmont Report—Ethical Principles and Guidelines for the Protection of Human Subjects of Research (1979)* provides the philosophical basis for federal regulatory requirements. It should be noted that the Common Rule in many ways "operationalizes" the principles of the Belmont Report.

1.3   The organization must assure compliance with applicable legal requirements, including state and local laws.

COMMENTARY on Standard 1.3: Organizations must comply with applicable federal regulations including the Common Rule, 45 CFR 46 (DHHS regulations), and 21 CFR 50 and 56 (FDA regulations) in all research conducted within the organization, regardless of the type of study, the source of funding, or the locale.

1.4   The organization must place the responsibility for the HRPP in an institutional official with sufficient standing and authority to ensure implementation and maintenance of the program.

COMMENTARY on Standard 1.4: An organization demonstrates that the protection of individuals studied in research is a priority by investing overall responsibility in an institutional official with demonstrated authority in the organization, with access to adequate resources to support the HRPP, and without conflicting responsibilities in other aspects of the organization's activities.

1.5   Individuals responsible for the HRPP must identify and minimize conflicts of interest, and/or competing interests, which may compromise the goals of the HRPP.

COMMENTARY on Standard 1.5: Institutional officials responsible for the HRPP should have clearly defined and institutionally supported responsibilities and authority in order to maximize their ability to achieve the goals stated in 1.5 without interference.

1.6   Any delegation of authority for the HRPP by the responsible institutional official (see 1.4 above) must be assigned to qualified individuals and documented in writing.

COMMENTARY on Standard 1.6: Any delegation of authority by the responsible institutional official to others requires serious and thoughtful attention. The institutional official must only delegate authority to qualified individuals and in situations that enhance the HRPP. Written documentation of delegation of authority is required to promote clear communication among the organization's constituencies and to establish an organizational record.

1.7   **The governance of the organization must assure the independence and credibility of the IRB(s).**

COMMENTARY on Standard 1.7: IRBs are one of several critical elements in an organization's HRPP. A successful HRPP requires that IRB members and chair(s) possess knowledge about ethical, regulatory, and institutional requirements. The IRB must be supported by the organization, which would necessarily exclude inappropriate influence by powerful officials, researchers, and potential funding sources. The IRB should have a clear mechanism for managing any influence that blocks or otherwise interferes with its functions.

1.8   **The organization must have conflict of interest policies and must enforce those policies to minimize real, potential, or perceived conflicts from interfering with the protection of individuals studied in research.**

COMMENTARY on Standard 1.8: Organizations must have a mechanism to address real or perceived conflicts of interest that could interfere with the protection of individuals studied in research. Organizational policies need to define conflicts of interest, provide mechanisms for disclosure of conflicts, establish a process for evaluating whether a conflict of interest may interfere with protection of the individuals studied in research, and institute actions to manage conflicts of interest determined to have the potential to interfere with that protection.

Organizations need to disseminate these policies to individuals responsible for the conduct of research involving humans and they need to determine what role the IRB should play in monitoring the application of these policies. The existence and enforcement of the organization's conflict of interest policies further demonstrates its commitment to place the protection of individuals involved in research above financial, professional, and other concerns.

1.9   **The organization must have and follow clearly written policies and procedures governing all human research. The policies and procedures must specify applicability. The policies and procedures must be re-**

viewed periodically and updated as necessary. The policies and procedures must be disseminated appropriately within the organization to
all staff involved with protection of individuals studied in research.

COMMENTARY on Standard 1.9: Mechanisms should be established
regarding when new policies and procedures are needed, and how existing policies and procedures should be reviewed and revised. Appropriate
intervals for this review and revision must be specified. New research
personnel must also be provided with this information and all staff must
be kept apprised of any changes.

1.10   The organization must assure that all personnel conducting or sup-
        porting human research or involved in the HRPP demonstrate and
        maintain sufficient knowledge of the protection of individuals studied
        in research appropriate to their role.

COMMENTARY on Standard 1.10: The organization must assure the
provision of acceptable educational activities for principal investigators,
other research personnel, IRB chairs, IRB members, IRB staff, appropriate institutional officials, and others in the organization as appropriate.

     The organization needs to assure that: (1) educational programs for
professional development in the area of protection of individuals studied
in research are appropriate to the investigator's role in the research; (2)
mechanisms exist to provide additional education as needed; (3) procedures exist for demonstrating the effectiveness of these activities; and (4)
individuals receive ongoing education at intervals determined appropriate
in consideration of their research endeavors. Appropriate procedures for
these individuals may involve attendance at courses, participation in
seminars, and/or completion of computer-based training. Supplemental
techniques such as performance feedback, monitoring, supervision, or
mentoring are also acceptable. (Please note that the NIH Required Policy
for IRB Review of Human Subjects Protocols in Grant Applications [No-
tice: OD-00-031: http://grants.nih.gov/grants/guide/notice-files/NOT-OD-
00-031.html] describes the minimum requirement for NIH grantees.)

1.11   The organization must establish the number of IRBs appropriate for
        the volume and types of human research that the IRBs review.

COMMENTARY on Standard 1.11: The trend in many research organizations is toward establishing more than one IRB. In large organizations conducting many research studies, it may be difficult for one IRB to
provide an adequate level of review of the protocols, particularly if they
are complex or originate from different disciplines (e.g., biomedical versus social and behavioral sciences). In determining the appropriate num-

ber of required IRBs, the organization should take into account the volume, complexity, and types of research it reviews. Organizations with multiple IRBs require additional thought and consideration to ensure that all human research subject protection issues are taken into account in a uniform manner.

1.12   The organization must provide sufficient and appropriate staff, space, equipment, finances, technology, and other resources for the HRPP.

COMMENTARY on Standard 1.12: The organization must determine what constitutes adequate resources. Input from the IRB(s) chairs, members, and staff is a critical ingredient in this determination (see further discussion of this issue in Section 2 of these Standards).

In addition to staffing needs, IRB administrative offices require enough space to maintain secure storage of records, to enable private communication, to provide current computer technology and support services, and to provide adequate space for meeting with investigators and IRB members.

1.13   The organization must recruit and retain IRB chair(s), members, and staff who have both experience and knowledge appropriate to their respective roles on the IRB team, and who represent all fields of science applicable to their organization.

COMMENTARY on Standard 1.13: The organization must both recruit and maintain a quality IRB by having high-caliber chairs, members, and staff. The organization's policies must foster the retention of individuals knowledgeable of and sensitive to the principles of the organization's human research protection program sufficient to assure continuity of high levels of performance. Appropriate and meaningful recognition, including but not limited to adjustments to compensation or organizational responsibilities, are central to the retention of knowledgeable and committed individuals.

1.14   The organization must have procedures for timely identification and dissemination of new information that may affect the HRPP, including laws, policies, and procedures, as well as emerging ethical and scientific issues.

1.15   The organization must have and follow written policies and procedures for addressing allegations and findings of non-compliance with the requirements of the HRPP, and management of research harms. The policies and procedures must be reviewed periodically and updated as necessary.

COMMENTARY on Standard 1.15: There must be a clear and public policy concerning identification and reporting of research harms and for the compassionate and efficient management of such events. These procedures must include a fair and reasonable process for all parties involved. Any accused individual should have the right to appear in person to defend himself/herself. The procedures should also include a mechanism that determines those violations serious enough to inform regulatory agencies and funding sources. The organization must have and follow a written policy that protects from retaliation those who in good faith report allegations of non-compliance. (Please note that the Office for Research Integrity's Notice of Proposed Rulemaking can be found at 65 Fed. Reg. 70830 (2000) and may be accessed by clicking on News on the ORI home page, http://ori.hhs.gov.)

1.16   **The organization must utilize a system for regularly assessing outcomes of and improving the performance of the HRPP. The system developed to examine results or outcomes of the HRPP's activities must also include the identification of problems, implementation of interventions, and measurement or evaluation of the effect of interventions.**

COMMENTARY on Standard 1.16: Performance evaluation and assessment of programmatic outcomes in other disciplines are well known and have become generally accepted as organizational best practice. Until now, they have neither been widely applied nor implemented by HRPPs.

Two reports, one by the Advisory Committee on Human Radiation Experiments (ACHRE) and the other by the DHHS Office of the Inspector General (OIG), concluded that an adequate system of human research protection "would require that the system be subjected to regular, periodic evaluations that are based on an examination of outcomes and performance and that include the perspective and experiences of research [subjects] as well as the research community." The OIG's Report recommended that IRBs be given more flexibility by the FDA and OPRR (now OHRP), with concomitantly a greater accountability for results by taking "concrete actions . . . to assess and verify the actual results of their efforts in protecting human subjects." The Report described a small number of creative efforts currently undertaken by some IRBs.

Persistent problems in human research protection and the changing nature of clinical research, public expectation, and organizational best practices have thus necessitated that the organization, IRBs, and investigators regularly evaluate their performance and assess outcomes. An organization seeking accreditation must propose its own methods/procedures for evaluating the performance of all aspects of the HRPP.

As performance evaluation of HRPPs, IRBs, and investigators becomes more routine around the United States, PRIM&R will publicize innovative programs that effectively address these organizational best practices.

1.17 The organization must provide evidence of programs, policies, or procedures for ongoing communication with representatives of the geographic and/or subject communities studied in research. These communication vehicles should provide for the ongoing discussion of commonalities and/or differences in research portfolios and agendas, goals of interest to either or both parties, and for the sharing of each other's values and concerns.

COMMENTARY on Standard 1.17: The organization must be aware of the customs and values in the respective research participant populations it serves, including legal requirements as appropriate. This awareness is especially important when research is being conducted or contemplated that involves individuals from that community (geographic, demographic, and cultural). For example, organizations conducting research involving Native Americans must understand and appreciate tribal concerns that influence the conduct of such research. Organizations whose IRBs are widely separated geographically from their investigators should detail the manner in which such potentially diverse communities will be engaged and involved.

Section 2—Institutional Review Boards (IRBs)

GENERAL COMMENTARY on Section 2: In fulfilling their mandate to protect the rights and welfare of individuals studied in research, IRBs are intended to be impartial reviewers of research studies. Their responsibilities include the review, approval, or disapproval of protocols, and the recommendation of protocol and/or consent modifications, all of which are designed to minimize the risks to the individuals to be recruited into the study.

2.1 The IRB(s) must comply with all applicable laws, regulations, and organizational policies and procedures.

COMMENTARY on Standard 2.1: See Standard 1.2

2.2 The IRB(s) must identify to the appropriate institutional officials the resources it requires.

COMMENTARY on Standard 2.2: The IRB staff, chair(s), and members constitute the relevant source of information concerning the needs for this component of the HRPP.

2.3 **Each IRB should be constituted to promote respect for its advice and counsel in safeguarding the rights and welfare of the individuals studied in research.**

COMMENTARY on Standard 2.3: The size of the organization and the extent of its research will determine the number of IRBs required. The type(s) of research reviewed by the IRB(s) (e.g., behavioral research, clinical trials, epidemiological research, and research involving vulnerable populations or minority groups) will influence membership requirements. Appropriate expertise of IRB members, chair(s), and staff is required to ensure an adequate review of protocols from varied disciplines. IRBs also need to recognize when consultant expertise is required.

2.4 **The IRB chair(s), members, and staff must possess sufficient respect within the organization and the leadership skills as a team sufficient to be an authority on the protection of individuals studied in research under the jurisdiction of the HRPP.**

COMMENTARY on Standard 2.4: The position of IRB chair is of singular importance, and requires commitment, knowledge, and the necessary leadership skills to serve as an effective steward. The responsibility of the chair should be vested in a highly credible member of the organization, as s/he will then be better able to engender respect for the authority of the IRB.

Attributes which are a measure of an effective IRB team include: (1) the ability to conduct meetings in an efficient, expeditious, and fair manner; (2) attentiveness to the details of applicable federal regulations and other legal and institutional requirements; (3) skillful facilitation of contextual interpretations and application of these requirements that will foster ethically and scientifically sound research involving human beings; (4) the ability to encourage dialogue in IRB meetings and within the organization; (5) respect for the contributions of all IRB members and staff, especially the contributions of the non-scientists and community representatives; (6) the confidence and courage to uphold IRB judgments, and (7) investment of adequate time, interest, and commitment by the chair, IRB members, IRB staff, researchers, and other interested individuals in the organization.

2.5   Knowledge, Skills, and Abilities
The IRB administrator, staff, chair(s), and Board members must possess and maintain knowledge, skills, and abilities appropriate to their role including:

General ethical principles and concepts underlying the conduct of research involving humans;

- **Applicable Federal, state, and local laws and regulations;**
- **Applicable HRPP and IRB policies and procedures;**
- **Role of the IRB(s) in the HRPP; and**
- **These Accreditation Standards**

COMMENTARY on Standard 2.5: Appropriate activities include education of new members, chair(s), and staff and continuing education for current staff, members, and chair(s) using performance feedback, mentoring, and monitoring techniques. These activities should be designed to ensure that IRB chairs, staff, and members know and apply the concepts and requirements in this Accreditation Standard.

Continuing education for an IRB team is particularly important in light of the breadth and depth of their expected knowledge base. Organizations should support the team's attendance at and/or participation in local, regional, and/or national meetings or programs on the protection of individuals studied in research.

Successful IRB administration requires a combination of a working knowledge of protection of those studied in research and skills in administration. Organizations should support appropriate training for IRB administration. This may include their attendance at and/or participation in meetings or programs on the protection of individuals studied in research, acquisition of topic-oriented journals/books, and/or professional development such as certification through the ARENA Council for Certification of IRB Professionals (CCIP).

2.6   In the review of protocols, the IRB must recognize when additional expertise is needed and must obtain that expertise (e.g., education in, or consultation on scientific, ethical, community representation, or other issues).

COMMENTARY on Standard 2.6: Some protocols may present new or special considerations beyond the scientific and ethical expertise of the IRB. The IRB should have and follow policies regarding inviting individuals with competence in special areas to assist in the review of protocols that require expertise in addition to that available within the IRB. These individuals can submit comments in writing and they may attend

IRB meetings in a non-voting capacity to present their findings. IRB procedures must specify in writing details regarding this process.

2.7 **IRBs must demonstrate systematic review of research protocols in order to assure that issues, regulations, and other applicable organizational policies and procedures relevant to the protection of individuals studied in research are consistently addressed.**

COMMENTARY on Standard 2.7: IRBs must determine, at a minimum, that all of the following criteria are satisfied: (1) Research risks are reasonable in relation to anticipated benefits; (2) Risks are minimized; (3) The selection of those in the population to be studied is equitable (the IRB should be particularly cognizant of the special problems of research involving vulnerable populations); (4) Informed consent is sought from research participants or their authorized representatives unless waived by the IRB; (5) Monitoring of data is appropriate to ensure safety; (6) Adequate provisions are made to protect privacy and maintain the confidentiality of research data, and (7) When vulnerability to coercion or undue influence may exist, additional safeguards are included in the study to protect the rights and welfare of individuals participating in the research.

2.8 **The IRB must ensure that consent documents are legible, understandable, well organized, and remain appropriate for the research population.**

COMMENTARY on Standard 2.8: Technical and legal language should be defined and stated in terminology that the research population can understand. Systematic feedback from coordinators, research participants, and investigators should be one method for implementing the assessment of the adequacy of the consent documents.

2.9 **The IRB must determine that the consent process is appropriate for the circumstances under which the research will be conducted.**

COMMENTARY on Standard 2.9: The entire process for obtaining informed consent must be considered in the IRB review including who, when, how, and any special circumstances pertinent to the process. The Principal Investigator (PI) of the study is responsible for all aspects of the consent process regardless of any special circumstances.

2.10 **The IRB must receive evidence that the investigator(s) is qualified through training, experience, and commitment of time and resources, to be responsible and appropriate for the planned research.**

COMMENTARY on Standard 2.10: The IRB should have policies that define acceptable evidence of the qualifications of the principal investigator and research team members as related to the specific protocol. These policies should also include provisions indicating how students and trainees are covered when the curriculum or training requires that research be accomplished.

2.11   **The IRB must have written policies and procedures pertaining to the following and which are appropriate and relevant to the types of research reviewed within the organization, including research involving special populations (children, persons who are decisionally impaired, the elderly, etc.) or certain types of research (e.g., social and behavioral research, drug washout studies, double-blinded placebo controlled studies, or research conducted in emergency circumstances).**

POLICIES REQUIRED OF ALL IRBs
(A) Initial IRB review of protocols

COMMENTARY on Standard 2.11 (A): IRB review of protocols must be complete and substantive. IRB members must receive sufficient information to make a determination of each review criterion.

(B) Substantive and meaningful continuing IRB review of protocols, including frequency of review and assuring that design and procedures continue to be appropriate and safe

COMMENTARY on Standard 2.11 (B): When conducting continuing review, all IRB members must receive sufficient information to allow the Board to pass judgment.

(C) Full review requirements (e.g., quorum requirements, asking IRB members who have conflicts of interest to recuse themselves, etc.)
(D) Requirements for the consent process, including the consent forms and their modifications
(E) Expedited review
(F) Exempt research
(G) If appropriate, procedures for the IRB's primary reviewer of the protocol
(H) Investigators' conflicts of interest

COMMENTARY on Standard 2.11 (H): In keeping with Standard 1.8, the IRB implements the organization's written conflicts of interest policies in regard to individuals studied in research. The IRB is responsible for determining whether any potential, real, or perceived conflicts of interest could affect the conduct of research under consideration or that could impact the safety of those individuals studied in research.

(I) Identification and reporting of adverse events (to the IRB and others as required)

(J) Procedures/rules for the review of PI's response(s) to IRB stipulations and recommendations

(K) Noncompliance by researchers or research personnel with protocol requirements and/or with IRB policies/procedures

(L) Suspensions or terminations of approvals

(M) Collaborative agreements (national and international)

(N) Reporting IRB findings to investigators, appropriate institutional officials, and appropriate federal or other regulatory agencies

(O) Advertisements and other recruitment-related materials

(P) Remuneration to research participants

(Q) Investigator record keeping and retention requirements

(R) Vulnerable populations

(S) Waiver of informed consent or of documentation of consent

(T) Any other relevant areas

POLICIES REQUIRED OF IRBs WITH SPECIAL INTERESTS

(A) Determining the regulatory status of an investigational device concerning the significance of the risk of the device, if needed

(B) Emergency use of IND compounds or other investigational interventions

(C) Grant review for certification of approval of research

(D) Any other relevant areas

2.12 The IRB protocol records/files must contain at least the below-listed information.

COMMENTARY on Standard 2.12: As the study file contains the details regarding the protocol and the review of that protocol, and as the file is subject to audit, it is necessary that the study file be complete, accessible, and archived. The IRB protocol records/files must contain at least the following information:

(A) A copy of the protocol, including approved consent documents and results of existing related information pertinent to the protocol

(B) Scientific evaluations reviewed by the IRB, if any

(C) Initial reviews

(D) Advertisements and other applicable recruitment materials

(E) Payments to be made to research participants (amount of payment, etc.)

(F) Continuing reviews and progress reports

(G) Adverse event reports with documentation of IRB review

(H) All correspondence (including electronic mail) with investigator(s), consultants, and others (institutional officials, sponsors, etc.) about the protocol.

(I) Statements of significant new findings provided to research participants

(J) Reports of non-compliance, if applicable

(K) Reports of deviations from approved protocols, if applicable

(L) Protocol modifications/amendments

(M) Suspensions or revocation of approval, if applicable

(N) Minutes relative to the protocol review and actions

(O) When applicable, the investigator's plan to communicate with representatives of the community from which individuals will be recruited in order to share the protocol and learn of community concerns, values, and expectations

2.13   IRB minutes, record keeping, and retention requirements.

COMMENTARY on Standard 2.13: IRB minutes are fundamental parts of its record keeping activities. The minutes, together with other IRB documents, should enable a reader who was not present at the meeting to determine how and with what justification(s) the IRB arrived at its decisions. The IRB must also have policies and procedures for retention of minutes and records.

(A)   The IRB meeting minutes must include at least the following information:

(1) Approval of minutes from the previous meeting;

(2) Attendance at meetings;

(3) Actions taken;

(4) Votes (including total number of members present) for, against, and abstaining, as well as names of abstainers, and reason for abstention, if appropriate;

(5) Documentation indicating change or loss of quorum throughout meeting;

(6) Summary of the discussion of issues and their resolution (including, when appropriate, minority reports);

(7) Basis for requiring changes, deferring, or disapproving protocols;

(8) Special findings (i.e., criteria for varying or altering consent requirements or risk categories for children and other vulnerable populations);

(9) Discussion of the need for a DSMB or other monitoring procedure(s) when applicable;

(10) When applicable, determination of significant/non-significant devices (for studies under the auspices of FDA investigational device regulations); and

(11) Requirements for frequency of continuing review, if more often than annually.

(B) The IRB files must include an IRB roster, members' qualifications, and organizational assurances including any relevant appendices, when appropriate. Documents should be archived for reference.

Section 3—Investigators and Other Research Personnel

GENERAL COMMENTARY on Section 3: The roles and responsibilities of investigators are influenced by the nature of the environment in which they conduct research (e.g., academic center, private practice/community setting, etc.) and by the type of research in which they are engaged. However, in all circumstances, investigators are an essential element in the protection of individuals enrolled in their respective research studies. Therefore, these Standards should apply irrespective of the manner in which the HRPP is constituted. The presence of an intelligent, informed, conscientious, compassionate, and responsible investigator is the best possible protection for all involved in the research process.

3.1 The investigator should understand and apply the underlying ethical principles as delineated in *The Belmont Report* when designing, or when evaluating already designed studies, and when conducting human research.

3.2 Investigators must put the rights, welfare, and safety of each individual studied in their research ahead of their professional, academic, financial, personal, or other interests.

COMMENTARY on Standard 3.2: The investigator's primary attention must be focused on the safety and welfare of the individuals who volunteer to participate and those included without their consent (e.g., use of preexisting data, etc.). Investigators must identify and avoid conflicts of interest that may interfere with the rights and welfare of research participants and the appropriate conduct of research.

3.3 Investigators must meet organizational requirements for conducting research with human subjects and comply with all applicable federal, state, and local regulations and guidelines dealing with the protection of individuals studied in research.

COMMENTARY on Standard 3.3: Investigators are responsible for the overall design, development, conduct, and analysis of the investigation, whether the investigator personally developed the protocol or if others prepared the protocol (e.g., as in a multicenter investigation). Investigators must have a collegial relationship with the IRB. Although many IRBs may have information manuals for investigators that cover the requirements, it is the investigator's responsibility to seek out and comply with those requirements even if the IRB does not overtly supply the supportive material.

3.4   Principal Investigators (PIs) must assure that all research involving human subjects is reviewed and approved by an IRB before study initiation and that it remains approved for the duration of the study.

COMMENTARY on Standard 3.4: The IRB should be consulted when questions arise regarding whether a given research activity constitutes human research. The IRB should be accorded the authority within the organization to determine what constitutes human research, as the IRB has specific expertise in making such decisions. The PI should be cognizant of the types of research that may be exempt from IRB review, or which can be processed by expedited review. This determination usually requires consultation with the IRB.

PIs must be familiar with the criteria for IRB review and approval indicated in Standard 2.7 and, at a minimum, be able to provide the IRB with this information as well as any continuing review information relevant to the research protocol.

Appropriate and continuing oversight of a research protocol by the PI includes orderly retention of research records, appropriate level of review, compilation, assessment, and appropriate reporting of adverse events. The PI has the responsibility for the prompt reporting to the IRB and sponsor(s) and appropriate federal agencies of any injuries, adverse events, or other unanticipated problems involving risks to subjects and others.

3.5   Principal Investigators must delegate responsibility only to individuals who they determine are qualified through training and experience for their role in the research.

COMMENTARY on Standard 3.5: The qualification of the PI to conduct the proposed research must be submitted to the IRB to provide adequate guidance for review. There should be a documented training and experience for the PI and PIs must assure that all research personnel involved in the protocol are qualified through training and experience to perform their role in the research.

3.6   Principal Investigators must conduct research in which individuals are studied only when supported by adequate resources including

staffing, time allocated by the staff to the research, funding, space, record-keeping capability, and back-up for adverse events.

3.7 **Principal Investigators should, when appropriate, communicate with potentially concerned sectors of the community or of the specific population to be recruited in their investigation.**

COMMENTARY on Standard 3.7: Discussions about research with prospective research participants and/or the community in which the research will be conducted is a regulatory requirement in some circumstances (e.g., FDA and other DHHS requirements for research conducted in emergency circumstances, etc.). However, investigators should be aware that community involvement in the design and conduct of some research studies may benefit research participants, researchers, and the community. For example, the likelihood of improving informed consent may be enhanced if the community has the opportunity to be included more directly in the decisions made by the organization. Addressing the concerns and values of the community early in the process can help engender a positive attitude in the community for the research organization and/or for the researcher.

3.8 **When appropriate, the investigator should explain to, and discuss with, the potential research participants their responsibilities to enhance their protection and to support the integrity of the investigation in ways which include:**
(A) Ensuring that research participants understand the risks and benefits of the study, and alternatives thereto;
(B) Ensuring that research participants know whom to contact when they feel they have been dealt with inappropriately;
(C) Ensuring that research participants know whom to contact on the research team if they believe that an adverse event has occurred; and
(D) Recognizing that the safety of research participants and the integrity of the research study are enhanced by ongoing and candid communications between research participant and researcher(s).

PUBLICATIONS CITED IN ACCREDITATION STANDARDS

U.S. Department of Health and Human Services, Office of Inspector General, "Institutional Review Boards: A Time for Reform," OEI-01-97-00193 (June 1998). Copies are available through the Boston office: (617) 565–1050, or the OIG Web site: http://www.dhhs.gov/progorg/oei

U.S. Department of Health and Human Services, Office of the Secretary, The National Commission for the Protection of Human Research Subjects, *The Belmont Report:*

Ethical Principles and Guidelines for the Protection of Human Subjects of Research (April 18, 1979). Copies are available at the following Web site: http://ohrp. ospophs.|dhhs.gov/humansubjects/guidance/belmont.htm

VA Human Research Protection Accreditation Program Draft Accreditation Standards

BACKGROUND

The Department of Veterans Affairs has contracted with NCQA to develop and implement an accreditation program for Veterans Affairs Medical Center (VAMC) Human Research Protection Programs (HRPPs). The purpose of the program is to strengthen the protections afforded human subjects of research at VAMCs through an ongoing program of independent, external review. The public must be assured that research is performed ethically and in the best interests of study volunteers to ensure its continued support for, and participation in, research studies. The VA has long held a set of policies governing the conduct of research, and in particular, the protection of human study participants. This program is the first to provide a routine, independent evaluation of VAMCs' compliance with these policies.

These draft standards for the accreditation of Veterans Affairs Medical Center (VAMC) Human Research Protection Programs (HRPPs) are being published for public comment. In June 2001, program standards will be finalized after analysis of public comments and results of pilot tests to be conducted in April and May, 2001. The resultant standards will be revised annually to reflect changes in VA policy and other applicable federal regulation.

These standards apply to VAMCs that operate their own IRBs, those that operate an IRB jointly with an affiliated university, and those that delegate IRB functions to the affiliated university's IRB. Standards include requirements for the oversight of affiliated IRBs. The VAMC retains responsibility for protecting human subjects of research even when it delegates the performance of some functions (e.g., IRB) to the affiliated university. All the standards for the performance of the IRB apply to the IRB, whether operated by the VAMC, the affiliated university, or jointly.

SOURCE OF STANDARDS

These draft standards were compiled from regulations and other applicable policies that apply to research conducted at VA medical facilities and by VA employees. The principal sources were:

- VA regulations at 38 CFR 16-17;
- DHHS regulations at 45 CFR 46;
- FDA regulations at 21 CFR 50, 56, 312, and 812;
- VA policy as documented in Chapter 9 of the M-3 manual;
- FDA Information Sheets;
- International Conference on Harmonisation Good Clinical Practice Guideline; and
- OHRP Compliance Activities: Common Findings and Guidance.

Accreditation standards may not necessarily match a specific regulation word-for-word. In general, if a regulation specifies an activity that must occur the standard reflects this fact, and focuses on measurable evidence that it occurred. Where allowed by a regulation, standards are flexible, for example, with respect to methods to be used to achieve a specified process or outcome. If a regulation has a specified intent, but does not specify how such intent shall be achieved, the required level of achievement, or other relevant details, standards were developed that are consistent with the expressed regulatory intent. Because these standards focus on VA research, they do not cover all regulations and policies pertaining to the conduct of international research, research involving children, fetuses, and prisoners, or genetic research.

ORGANIZATION OF THE STANDARDS

In this document unless otherwise specified, the term "standards" encompasses the rationale, standards, requirements, and elements, inclusively. The standards are organized into the following six domains:

1. Institutional Responsibilities;
2. IRB Structure and Operation;
3. Consideration of Risks and Benefits;
4. Subject Recruitment and Selection;
5. Privacy and Confidentiality; and
6. Informed Consent.

Each of the six domains of standards includes a statement of rationale. Following in hierarchical fashion, are standards, requirements, and elements that detail the performance expectations of the VAMC HRPP. The standards are organized to indicate a chain of activity, from policy and procedure (suggesting intent), through results (documented demonstration that the intent is being met and the desired outcome achieved). Each standard may be composed of one or several requirements.

Each requirement contains many specific elements that provide detail and dimension to the requirement. Standards pertain to the following areas:

- Policies and procedures;
- Implementation of required activities;
- Performance of activities to demonstrate the HRPP is achieving required results (quality assurance and improvement); and
- Required results.

Standards identify the allowable sources of evidence, and methods for the evaluation of evidence, to determine whether or not a particular standard has been met. While many data sources may be listed for a requirement, they are generally listed as alternative sources. That is, a VAMC need not demonstrate compliance with a requirement in each and every data source listed; rather, it must demonstrate compliance in at least one data source (and not contradict the finding in others). Interviews are the exception and will be used only to clarify and confirm information from other sources. Data sources listed are intended to provide information about different aspects of performance (generally reflected in the different elements). For example, a requirement may include data sources such as policies and procedures, as well as IRB protocol files. In this instance, the surveyor will look for evidence that the HRPP has a policy or procedure governing an issue, and will look in a sample of protocol files to assess whether the policy has been implemented effectively.

The accreditation survey will result in one of four outcomes, as documented in the draft Accreditation Outcome Table below. Depending on their performance, Human Research Protection Programs can achieve Full Accreditation, Conditional Accreditation, Probational Accreditation, or No Accreditation. Each accreditation outcome brings with it a set of actions by NCQA as well as VA offices. These actions include, for example, follow-up oversight by NCQA, VA Office of Research and Development requirements for, and restrictions on, starting new research or continuing research, and VA Office of Research Compliance and Assurance follow-up, remedial action, and training. Please note that NCQA can only address its own actions and policies related to each outcome.

TABLE C-1 Draft Accreditation Outcomes and Remedial Action

Outcome	Description	Criteria	Programmatic Outcome	Actions by ORCA	Actions by ORD	Actions by Accreditor
Full	Meets all standards at acceptable level.	Score above xx points on 100-point scale; *performance meets all threshold standards.*	Research continues. Resurvey in 3 years.	Reviews accreditation report. [Note: May independently comment or request additional information from the VAMC.]	Reviews accreditation report. [Note: May independently comment or request additional information from the VAMC.]	Resurvey in 3 years.
Conditional	Meets most standards at acceptable level.	Score between yy and xx points on 100-point scale; *performance meets all threshold standards.*	Research may proceed. Submit Remediation Action Plan (RAP) to accreditor, ORCA, and ORD within 30 days.	Reviews accreditation report. [Note: May independently comment or request additional information from the VAMC. Monitors performance against RAP via periodic VAMC reporting at least until Full Accreditation is achieved. May require education and development (TED) program.]	Reviews accreditation report. [Note: May independently comment or request additional information from the VAMC. Monitors performance against RAP via periodic VAMC reporting at least until Full Accreditation is achieved.]	Monitors performance against periodic VAMC reporting at least until Full Accreditation is achieved. Follow-up survey may advance to Full Accreditation when RAP is fully implemented. Resurvey in 3 years (from date of original accreditation determination).

| Probational | Meets some standards at acceptable level, but inadequate performance on many others. | Score between zz and yy points on 100-point scale; *performance meets all threshold standards*. | No new projects may be initiated until all deficiencies are corrected. Submit RAP to accreditor, ORCA, and ORD within 30 days. | Reviews accreditation report [Note: May independently comment or request additional information from the VAMC. Monitors performance against RAP via periodic VAMC reporting at least until Full Accreditation is achieved. May require TED program. Consider ORCA site visit.] | Reviews accreditation report. [Note: May independently comment or request additional information from the VAMC. Monitors performance against RAP via periodic VAMC reporting at least until Full Accreditation is achieved. In addition, withhold funding for new projects and may withdraw funding for current projects until at least Conditional Accreditation is achieved.] | Follow-up survey required to advance to Conditional Accreditation. Resurvey in 1 year (from date of Accreditation upgrade to Conditional). |

Continued

TABLE C-1 *Continued*

Outcome	Description	Criteria	Programmatic Outcome	Actions by ORCA	Actions by ORD	Actions by Accreditor
Not Accredited	Fails to meet basic accreditation standards.	Score below zz points on 100-point scale; OR unacceptable performance on one or more threshold standards.	All research must cease until corrections are made. A patient already enrolled in studies may continue only if that is in the subject's best interest. No new subjects may be enrolled and no new projects may be started. Submit RAP to accreditor, ORCA, and ORD within 30 days.	Reviews accreditation report [Note: May independently add comments or request additional information from VAMC. Monitors performance against RAP via periodic VAMC reporting at least until Full Accreditation is achieved. May require TED program. Consider ORCA site visit.]	Reviews accreditation report. [Note: May independently add comments or request additional information from the VAMC. Monitors performance against RAP periodic VAMC reporting at least until Full Accreditation is achieved. Withdraw funding for all research (except amounts required to assure patient safety) until at least Probational Accreditation is achieved.]	Decides when to determine if site can advance to Probational Accreditation. Resurvey in 1 (one) year (from date of Accreditation upgrade to Probational).

NOTE: At the accreditor's discretion, a site may not need to have a follow-up survey to move out of Conditional status to Full Accreditation. Rev. 12/21/00

OPERATION OF ACCREDITATION PROGRAM

VAMCs to be accredited will submit documents to demonstrate their compliance with accreditation program standards. A team of certified surveyors will visit each VAMC to be accredited. Surveyors will verify the VAMC's compliance with each standard and record their assessments in a structured report. The VAMC will be allowed to comment on the report's accuracy. The Program Accreditation Committee will review the surveyors' report and any VAMC comments, and issue an accreditation decision.

PROGRAM COMPONENTS UNDER DEVELOPMENT

Work is still underway to finalize data collection methods and protocol sampling strategies. These will be formalized in guidelines for surveyors. Sampling issues under consideration include how many protocols to sample and how to stratify samples to provide meaningful information about issues that present infrequently in some institutions. In addition to work on the sampling strategies, work is underway to determine the scoring of elements and requirements, including those that are applicable only in some instances (e.g., requirements relating to planned emergency research). First-year scoring will be more lenient than scoring in future years, when it will be possible to provide more advance notice of standards. Finally, the threshold scores required to achieve each accreditation outcome will be determined after each element's and requirement's relative weight has been determined. Comments on sampling and scoring are invited along with comments on the standards, requirements, elements, data sources, and review methods presented.

DEFINITIONS

ADVERSE EVENT (AE) Any untoward medical occurrence that does not necessarily have a causal relationship with treatment. An AE can be any unfavorable and unintended sign, symptom, or disease.

AFFILIATE'S HUMAN RESEARCH PROTECTION PROGRAM The HRPP of a VAMC's academic affiliate. See HRPP.

CERTIFICATE OF CONFIDENTIALITY Where data are being collected from subjects about sensitive issues (such as illegal behavior, alcohol or drug use, or sexual practices or preferences), researchers can obtain an advance grant of confidentiality from the Public Health Service that will provide protection even against a subpoena for research data.

FDA FORM 3454 The financial disclosure form required by the FDA to reveal/identify any potential financial conflict of interest that an investigator(s), sub-investigator(s), or their spouse and children may have that is applicable to the submission of marketing applications for human drug, biological product, or device for each covered study.

FEDERALWIDE ASSURANCE (FWA) An agreement or contract between the institution and OHRP, on behalf of the Secretary, HHS, stipulating the method(s) by which the organization will protect the welfare of research subjects in accordance with the regulations. The Assurance, approval of which is a condition of receipt of DHHS support for research involving human subjects, spells out the organization's responsibilities for meeting the requirements of 45 CFR 46. The FWA replaces all other previous forms of assurance (i.e., MPA, SPA, etc.).

FOOD AND DRUG ADMINISTRATION (FDA) The federal agency responsible for the regulation of food, drugs, and cosmetics, including the human subject research performed for FDA-regulated articles.

HUMAN RESEARCH PROTECTION PROGRAM (HRPP) The systematic and comprehensive approach by an organization to ensure human subject protection in all research. The implementation of any part of the program may be delegated to specific committees, individuals, or entities (i.e., academic affiliate or another VAMC) by the organization.

HUMAN SUBJECT A living individual about whom a research investigator (whether professional or student conducting research) obtains data through intervention or interaction with the individual or identifiable information.

INSTITUTION The individual VAMC. The institution retains ultimate responsibility for human subject protection in research conducted at their facility and/or by their staff.

INSTITUTIONAL REVIEW BOARD (IRB) An independent committee comprised of scientific and non-scientific members established according to the requirements outlined in Title 38, part 16 (same as Title 45, part 46 and Title 21, part 56) of the U. S. Code of Federal Regulations.

INVESTIGATIONAL DEVICE EXEMPTION (IDE) The process by which the FDA permits a device that otherwise would be required to comply with a performance standard or to have premarket approval to be shipped lawfully for the purpose of conducting investigations of that device.

INVESTIGATIONAL NEW DRUG APPLICATION (IND) The process by which new drugs or biologics, including the new use of an approved drug, are registered with the FDA for administration to human subjects. An IND number is assigned by the FDA to the drug or biologic for use in tracking.

INVESTIGATOR (Principal investigator) An individual who conducts an investigation, that is, under whose immediate direction research is conducted, or, in the event of an investigation conducted by a team of individuals, is the responsible leader of that team.

INVESTIGATOR/SPONSOR A term defined in the FDA regulations as an individual with responsibility for initiating and conducting a research study.

LEGALLY AUTHORIZED REPRESENTATIVE An individual, judicial, or other body authorized under applicable law to consent on behalf of a prospective subject to the subject's participation in the procedure(s) involved in research.

MEDWATCH The FDA Medical Products Reporting Program, is an initiative designed both to educate all health professionals about the critical importance of being aware of, monitoring for, and reporting adverse events and problems to FDA and/or the manufacturer and to ensure that new safety information is rapidly communicated to the medical community, thereby improving patient care. The purpose of the MedWatch program is to enhance the effectiveness of postmarketing surveillance of medical products as they are used in clinical practice and to rapidly identify significant health hazards associated with these products.

MEMORANDUM OF UNDERSTANDING (MOU) A legal agreement outlining the details of the relationship between organizations, including the responsibilities of each. Such an agreement is used by the VAMC to delineate the terms and conditions under which it may utilize another entity's IRB.

MINIMAL RISK The probability and magnitude of harm or discomfort anticipated in the research are not greater in and of themselves than those ordinarily encountered in daily life or during the performance of routine physical or psychological examinations or tests.

MULTIPLE PROJECT ASSURANCE (MPA) An agreement or contract between the institution and OPRR, on behalf of the Secretary, HHS, stipulating the method(s) by which the organization will protect the welfare of research subjects in accordance with the regulations. The Assurance, approval of which is a condition of receipt of DHHS support for research involving human subjects, spells out the organization's responsibilities for meeting the requirements of 45 CFR 46. MPAs will be replaced by FWAs.

POLICY A principle or course of action to guide decision-making.

PROCEDURE See Standard Operating Procedure (SOP).

PROTOCOL A plan that includes, at minimum, the objectives, rationale, design, methods, and other conditions for the conduct of a research study.

PROTOCOL FILE The documents maintained by the IRB administration containing the protocol, investigator's brochure, IRB/investigator communications, and all other supporting materials.

QUALITY IMPROVEMENT (QI) The effort to assess and improve the level of performance of a program or institution. QI includes quality assessment and implementation of corrective actions to address any deficiencies identified.

RESEARCH A systematic investigation, including development, testing, and evaluation, designed to develop or contribute to generalizable knowledge.

SAFETY REPORTS (IND/IDE) Written reports from sponsors notifying the FDA and all participating investigators of any adverse experience associated with the use of a drug that is both serious and unexpected.

SERIOUS ADVERSE EVENT (SAE) Any event that results in death, a life-threatening situation, hospitalization or prolonged hospitalization, persistent or significant disability/incapacity, or a congenital anomaly/birth defect. SAEs require reporting to the sponsor and the IRB.

SPONSOR Any person or entity who takes responsibility for and initiates a clinical study. The sponsor may be an individual, pharmaceutical company, device manufacturer, governmental agency, academic institution, private organization, or other organization.

STANDARD OPERATING PROCEDURE (SOP) A formalized established series of steps for the uniform performance of a function or activity.

UNEXPECTED ADVERSE EVENT Any adverse event that has not previously been observed (e.g., included in the investigator brochure).

VULNERABLE SUBJECTS Individuals whose willingness to volunteer in a research study may be unduly influenced or coerced and individuals with limited autonomy.

TABLE C-2 INSTITUTIONAL RESPONSIBILITIES

Rationale

Each institution engaged in research involving human subjects is responsible for ensuring the rights, safety, and well-being of those recruited to participate in research activities. It is also responsible for assuring that investigators and their staffs understand and comply with standards for the ethical conduct of research. These broad responsibilities can be met through three institutional actions: developing a Human Research Protections Program to monitor, evaluate, and improve the protection of human research subjects; establishing and/or designating an Institutional Review Board to review research following federal and institutional requirements; and educating staff involved in research about their ethical responsibility to protect research participants. This standard outlines the responsibilities of institutions that conduct human subjects research.

KEY for Regulatory Guidance

CFR = Code of Federal Regulations
M-3, Part 1 = The Veterans Affairs Manual, Chapter 9
VA MPA = Veterans Affairs Multiple Project Assurance Contract
IRB-GB = OPRR IRB Guidebook
FDA-IS = FDA Information Sheets
FDA-IS, (CL) = Appendix H: Self-Evaluation Checklist for IRBs
FDA-IS, (FAQ) = Frequently Asked Question
FDA-IS, (ICG) = The Guide to Informed Consent
FDA-IS, (CR) = Continuing Review After Study Approval
ICH-GCP = International Conference on Harmonization, Good Clinical Practice Guidelines
OHRP CFG = OHRP Compliance Activities: Common Findings and Guidance for 9/1/2000

IR 1 The institution has a systematic and comprehensive program, Human Research Protection Program (HRPP), with dedicated resources to ensure the rights, safety, and well-being of human research subjects in relation to their participation in research activities.

Requirement	Element	Data Source	Method
1.A. The institution has a written description of (or plan for) its human research protection program (HRPP) appropriate for the volume and nature of the human subject research conducted at the institution.	1.A.1. The description includes: 1.A.1.1. A statement of principles concerning the protection of human research subjects. 1.A.1.2. The institutional officer accountable for the HRPP.	HRPP plan HRPP employee list, including time allocation (i.e., FTE)	Review documents for presence of each requirement of the standard
	1.A.1.3. The organizational structure, process, roles, and responsibilities for making policy to protect human research subjects.	FWA, MPA, or other assurance	
Regulation/Source	1.A.1.4. A process to identify and incorporate changes in VA and federal regulations and policies into the HRPP.	Relevant institutional or IRB policies and procedures	
38 CFR 16.103 M-3, Part 1, 9.07 VA MPA	1.A.1.5. A description of the types of research to be undertaken and the classes of subjects to be regularly included.	IRB and other committee charters, organizational charts	
45 CFR 46.103 45 CFR 46.107(e) OHRP CFG IRB-GB, (I)(B) IRB-GB, (II)(ii) FDA-IS, (FAQ)(I)	1.A.1.6. The description specifically addresses whether vulnerable persons will be regularly included in research and whether additional protections for vulnerable persons are needed in accordance with VA policy. 1.A.1.7. The institution has one or more of the following arrangements for an IRB:	Current Memoranda of Understanding or current written agreements for designated IRB(s)	
45 CFR 46.103b(2) M-3, Part 1, 9.07(b) IRB-GB, (I)(B) 45 CFR 46.103b(4) OHRP CFG (A)(1), (B), (C),(D),(E)	1.A.1.7.1. The institution sponsors its own IRB. 1.A.1.7.2. The institution has a written arrangement with a regional VA IRB or another VA IRB. 1.A.1.7.3. The institution has a written arrangement with an affiliated medical or dental school or university. 1.A.1.8. The HRPP description includes a resource plan or budget and a defined process for allocating resources. 1.A.1.9. The HRPP description specifies the role, organizational structure, and functions of the R&D Committee.	HRPP budget, HRPP resource analysis	

the IRB(s) and other committees and individuals with responsibilities for protecting human subjects in research. 1.A.1.10. The HRPP description specifies the education and training requirements for individuals with roles in the HRPP, including: 1.A.1.10.1. VA HQ education and training requirements. 1.A.1.10.2. Any additional institutional requirements. 1.A.1.11. The HRPP includes policies and procedures to address complaints, allegations, and findings of noncompliance with institution policies. 1.A.1.12. The HRPP description includes a plan for monitoring program effectiveness and applicability, including monitoring compliance with applicable VA, federal, state, and local policies and regulations.		Review of the mechanism used by the institution, annual review process, and the presence of an information system for tracking of IRB data.
1.B. The institution provides sufficient resources for the HRPP and its IRB(s). *Regulation/Source* 38 CFR 16.103 M-3 Part 1, 9.07(b) 45 CFR 46.103(b)(2) IRB-GB, (I)(B)	1.B.1. To ensure sufficient resources the institution does the following: 1.B.1.1. The institution has a mechanism for determining resource needs for the HRPP and its IRB(s) that includes staff, equipment, materials, and space. 1.B.1.2. The institution annually reviews those resource needs based on the type of research being conducted, the volume of research being reviewed, and feedback from IRB members and staff. 1.B.2. The institution has an information system, database, or log capable of tracking: 1.B.2.1. Research proposal status. 1.B.2.2. QI data.	HRPP and budget; interviews with HRPP staff (R&D and IRB staff); observation of equipment, materials, and document storage facilities.

148

| 1.C. The Institution maintains and supports a current and approved Federalwide Assurance (FWA) with OHRP and/or an assurance in accordance with current VA regulations that includes its principles and guidelines for protecting human subjects.

Regulation/Source
38 CFR 16.103
VA MPA
45 CFR 46.103(b–f)
IRB-GB, (I)(B)
FDA-IS, (FAQ)(I)
OHRP Requirements | The institution demonstrates its maintenance and support of a Federalwide Assurance in the following ways:
1.C.1. The institution is operating under an approved assurance.
1.C.2. The institution has policies and procedures in place governing the conduct of the assurance.
1.C.3. The institution adheres to any conditions or restrictions to the approved assurance and communicates these to the IRB(s) and investigators.
1.C.4. The institution registers its IRB(s) as required under an OHRP Federalwide Assurance.
1.C.5. The institution holds MOUs with IRBs that it uses. These IRBs must be registered as required by federal regulations.
1.C.6. The IRB(s) provides to the investigator a form indicating IRB approval. For VA protocols, it shall be the form VA 10-1223.
1.C.7. The institution updates its assurances and IRB registration as required by OHRP and in accordance with VA policies.
1.C.8. The institution identifies the responsible official for the assurance.
   1.C.8.1. In VA facilities, the Medical Center Director/CEO is the responsible official. | Assurance Certifications, review of approved grant applications, HRPP policies and procedures

Review for current, approved assurance and certifications (not expired or suspended, dated within 3 years of date of application) |

1.D. If the institution uses the IRB(s) of a VA regional university system, affiliated university, or another VA facility, the arrangement is specified in writing and the institution conducts oversight activities. *Regulation/Source* 38 CFR 16.103 M-3, Part 1, 9.07 VA MPA 45 CFR 46.103	1.D.1. For each such arrangement, there is a memorandum of Understanding (MOU). The MOU describes: 1.D.1.1. Specific requirements for the membership and operation of the IRB to review VA research in compliance with VA regulations. 1.D.1.2. The respective responsibilities of the institution and the designated IRB for human subject protection. 1.D.1.3. The scope of activities delegated to the IRB. 1.D.1.4. The method, frequency, and nature of reporting to the institution. 1.D.1.5. The process by which the institution evaluates the IRB's performance. 1.D.1.6. The remedies, including revocation of the designation, available to the institution if the designated IRB does not fulfill its obligations. 1.D.2. The institution conducts sufficient oversight of designated IRB(s). The institution: 1.D.2.1. Evaluates the designated IRB's capacity to perform the designated activities prior to designation. 1.D.2.2. Evaluates the designated IRB's charter, policies, procedures, and membership annually. 1.D.2.3. Evaluates regular reports as specified in 1.4 above. 1.D.2.4. Evaluates annually whether the designated IRB is in compliance with current VA, federal, and other regulations and guidance.	Current Memorandum of Understanding Minutes of R&D Committee, IRB minutes reviewed by R&D Committee, and reports from designated IRB on performance (prior to MOU execution) Designated IRB charter, policies, membership reviewed and approved annually Reports on current performance reviewed	MOU for each arrangement has the requirements of the standard Frequency of R&D review of IRB QI Reports on the effectiveness of designated IRBs evaluate the requirements of the standard documentation of evaluation results

1.E The institution periodically reviews the composition of its IRB(s)	The institution's periodic review of its IRB consists of the following:	Review for the presence of institutional review meeting the requirements of the standard.
	1.E.1. The IRB(s) and the membership of the IRB(s) are appropriate given the research being reviewed.	
Regulation/Source 38 CFR 16.103 M-3 Part 1,9.07(b) 45 CFR 46.103(b)(2) IRB-GB, (I)(B)	1.E.2. The IRB(s) includes representatives with an interest in or experience with vulnerable populations involved in research, either as members or ad hoc consultants.	Committee meeting minutes Institutional communication Institutional procedure
	1.E.3. Determination that the qualifications and experience of the Chair and members are appropriate for the research being reviewed.	IRB membership lists at specific intervals
	1.E.4. The IRB membership meets VA and Federal standards.	
1.F. The institution has policies and procedures to identify and manage institutional, IRB member, and investigator conflicts of interest with research conducted at the institution.	The institution's policies and procedures include:	Policies and procedures
	1.F.1. Identification and management of financial conflict of interest of the institution.	
	1.F.2. Identification and management of financial conflict of interest of IRB members.	Review of policies and procedures on conflict of interest
	1.F.3. Identification and management of financial conflict of interest of investigators.	Review of disclosure documentation
Regulation/Source ICH-GCP 5.1 21 CFR 54		FDA Form 3454 Disclosure documents IRB minutes Review of IRB minutes for IRB member disclosure of conflict of interest
1.G. The institution provides a system enabling research subjects to ask questions or to voice concerns or complaints.	The institution has the following procedures in place:	Individual responsible and procedure description
	1.G.1. The institution designates a specific individual with the responsibility to respond to questions, concerns, or complaints.	Complaints
	1.G.1.1. The name and telephone number of the individual(s) are included in all consent forms.	Review the procedure description and reports or data on questions, concerns, and complaints
Regulation/Source 38 CFR 16.116(a)(7)	1.G.2. The institution ensures a response to each question, concern, or complaint and that action is taken, as needed	

Standard	Elements	Evidence	Review
M3, Part 1, Appendix–Procedures for Obtaining Informed Consent (10) 45 CFR 46.116(a)(7) 21 CFR 50.25(a)(7)	1.G.3. The institution implements its policies and procedures to address complaints, allegations, and findings of noncompliance with HRPP and IRB policies.		
1.H. The institution ensures that the use of investigational products in research with human subjects is carried out consistent with VA and federal regulations. *Regulation/Source* M3, Part 1, 9.15 21 CFR 312 21 CFR 812	The use of investigational products or devices is subject to the following institutional processes: 1.H.1. The institution's Pharmacy Service has policies and procedures for the storage, security, and dispensing of investigational test articles that follow federal regulations and are in accordance with VA policy. 1.H.2. The institution ensures that Pharmacy Service conducts audits of its compliance with policies and procedures regarding the use of investigational test articles and uses the results for quality improvement purposes. 1.H.3. The institution has policies and procedures for the storage, security, and dispensing of investigational devices that follow federal regulations and are in accordance with VA policy. 1.H.4. The institution ensures that audits of compliance with policies and procedures are conducted regarding the use of investigational devices and uses the results for quality improvement.	Pharmacy Service policies and procedures for investigational drugs. Results of audits or reports of compliance. Institutional	Review for policies and procedures that address the requirements of the standard Documentation of audit results and evidence of interventions when noncompliance is identified
1.I. The institution's plan for monitoring program effectiveness and conducting quality improvement is implemented and includes measuring, assessing, and improving compliance with HRPP policies, assurances,	1.I.1. A designated committee or individual has responsibility for ensuring that the HRPP plan is operational. Specific responsibilities include: 1.I.1.1. The implementation of HRPP policy. 1.I.1.2. The review and evaluation of the reports and results of monitoring compliance assessment and quality improvement activities. 1.I.1.3. The implementation of needed actions and follow-	HRPP compliance plan Job description(s) HRPP policies and procedures	Review of compliance plan for evidence of requirements Review of job descriptions for evidence of roles in HRPP Review of policies and procedures for evidence of require-

and other requirements for the protection of human subjects in research. *Regulation/Source* 38 CFR 16.103 M3, Part 1, 9.09(f) VA MPA 45 CFR 46.103 IRB-GB, (I)(B)(D) FDA-IS, (FAQ)(III)(24)	up on actions, as appropriate. 1.1.1.4. The documentation of its decisions and actions through dated and signed contemporaneous committee minutes. Or in the case of an individual, written documentation to record and communicate the individual's decisions and actions. 1.1.2. The institution monitors its performance in protecting human subjects. 1.1.3. The institution monitors the performance of the VA or the affiliate IRB(s). Monitoring includes the following areas: 1.1.3.1. Evaluation of the informed consent process. 1.1.3.2. Evaluation of the content and accuracy of informed consent forms. 1.1.3.3. Evaluation of research proposal risk and benefit including designation of minimal risk when appropriate. 1.1.3.4. Evaluation of special considerations and protections for vulnerable or potentially vulnerable populations. 1.1.3.5. Evaluation of privacy and confidentiality protections. 1.1.3.6. Evaluation of continuing review of approved research. 1.1.3.7. Use of expedited review, emergency review, or other procedures requiring review of less than the full IRB. 1.1.3.8. Granting exemption from federal requirements for IRB review. 1.1.3.9. Granting waivers for documentation of informed consent. 1.1.3.10. Granting waivers of any informed consent requirements. 1.1.3.11. Continuing review of safety and monitoring. 1.1.4. The institution monitors the performance of investigators. Monitoring includes the following areas: 1.1.4.1. Use of approved consent forms and procedures. 1.1.4.2. Obtaining consent prior to initiating any research-	ment to monitor HRPP plan HRPP Committee minutes or individual correspondence Monitoring or compliance reports	Review of minutes from the committee with designated responsibility for HRPP monitoring for review of monitoring in the areas required by the standards (or correspondence of designated individual) Review for the presence of a report or documentation of monitoring in the areas required by the standards

1.1.4.3. Reporting of all required safety issues and protocol deviations.

1.1.4.4. Adherence to HRPP policies and IRB approved protocols and conditions.

1.1.5. The institution monitors its responsiveness and reporting about subject questions, concerns, and complaints. Monitoring includes:

1.1.5.1. Review of data on questions, concerns, and complaints for reporting and quality improvement purposes.

1.1.6. The institution makes improvements to the HRPP based on performance monitoring results.

IR 2 The institution is responsible for educating institutional staff involved in research on their responsibility to protect the rights, safety, and well-being of human research subjects and holding them accountable for human subject protections.

Requirement	Elements	Data Source	Method
2.A. The institution is responsible for ensuring that research investigators, research staff, IRB members, and other individuals with responsibility for human subject protection have completed required training in human subject protection.	The institution's responsibilities for training investigators and staff in human subject protection include the following:	Policies, forms, checklists, and related HRPP and IRB materials	Review of materials requirements and the method of communication of HRPP and IRB
	2.A.1. The institution has information on HRPP requirements and IRB requirements.		
	2.A.2. The institution communicates information on HRPP and IRB requirements to investigators and other individuals with human subject protection responsibility and makes it readily available.		
Regulation/Source	2.A.3. The institution has a description of the type and scope of human subject protection education and training that meets VA and other regulatory requirements.		
VA MPA			
OHRP Requirements	2.A.4. The institution ensures that investigators and other individuals have received education and training appropriate to their roles.	Training programs and materials	Training log reflects training for all investigators. The institution
IRB-GB, (I)(B)		Description of educational and training requirements	has taken steps to train staff where gaps exist
	2.A.5. The institution periodically evaluates the training and certification status of research investigators, IRB members, and other individuals with responsibility for human subject protection.	Training log for the past year	
		Database on training certification	
	2.A.6. The institution has taken steps to train staff where identified gaps exist in education and training.	List of all investigators, IRB members, and HRPP staff from the past year	

2.B. The institution provides proper guidance to investigators regarding development of consent forms and conduct of the consent process. *Regulation/Source* IRB-GB, ((I)(B) FDA-IS, (ICG) M-3 21 CFR 50.23(a) 21 CFR 50.24	The institution provides guidance in the following areas: 2.B.1. Model consent forms. 2.B.2. Memoranda or other communications to investigators concerning conduct of the consent process, documentation of consent, and content of consent forms. 2.B.3. Provision of mandatory training on the consent process. 2.B.4. IRB policies and procedures. 2.B.5. New VA, federal, and local regulations, when appropriate.	Communications to investigators, training logs, model consent forms, guidance materials, etc. HRPP and IRB policies and procedures	Surveyors assess the completeness of materials.

156

TABLE C-3 INDIVIDUAL IRB STRUCTURE AND OPERATIONS

Rationale

Institutional Review Boards (IRB) are the administrative bodies established to protect the rights and welfare of human research subjects through prospective and concurrent review of research. IRB structure, composition, and function must be sufficient to allow for thorough and expert review of research to ensure that subjects are adequately protected. This standard contains the requirements for IRB membership and processes to provide adequate supervision of research.

KEY:

CFR = Code of Federal Regulations
M-3, Part 1 = The Veterans Affairs Manual, Chapter 9
IRB-GB = OPRR IRB Guidebook
FDA-IS = FDA Information Sheets
FDA-IS, (CL) = Appendix H: A Self-Evaluation Checklist for IRBs
FDA-IS, (FAQ) = Frequently Asked Questions
FDA-IS, (ICG) = The Guide to Informed Consent
FDA-IS, (CR) = Continuing Review After Study Approval
FDA-IS, (SR/NSR) = Significant Risk and Nonsignificant Risk Medical Device Studies
ICH-GCP = International Conference on Harmonization, Good Clinical Practice Guideline
OHRP-CFG = Office of Human Research Protection Compliance Activities: Common Findings and Guidance 9/1/2000
HHSIGR = HHS Inspector General's Report

IRB 1 The IRB's structure and composition are appropriate to the amount and nature of research reviewed and meet regulatory requirements.

Requirement	Element	Data Source	Method
1.A. The IRB maintains, or has access to, information about each IRB member. *Regulation/Source* 38 CFR 16.103(b)(3) 38 CFR 16.115 (a)(5) M-3, Part 1, 9.09 (g)(1)(e) 45 CFR 46.103(b)(3) 45 CFR 46.115a(5) 21 CFR 56.115(a)(5) IRB-GB, (I)(B) FDA-IS, (CL)(VI) ICH-GCP, (3.21)	Information about each IRB member includes the following: 1.A.1. Name and address. 1.A.2. Earned degrees. 1.A.3. Representative capacity (e.g., physician, non-scientist, ethicist, community member, etc.). 1.A.4. Indications of experience, such as board certifications, licensures, certifications, etc. 1.A.5. For community members, past or present association with the VA (including academic affiliates) or its employees. 1.A.6. Statement of financial and other interests which may constitute a conflict of interest. 1.A.7. Documentation of training in human subject protection. 1.A.8. Documentation of the voting status of each member. 1.A.9. Documentation of alternate status.	Files maintained by the institution on each IRB member including but not limited to: curriculum vitae; disclosure documentation; copies of training certificates	Review of IRB files shows compliance with requirements for current and past IRB members for the past one year

Standard	Requirements	Documentation	Verification
1.B. The IRB consists of the appropriate number, type, and diversity of members. *Regulation/Source* 38 CFR 16.107 (a)(b)(c)(d) M-3, Part 1, 9.08(a) 45 CFR 46.107 (a)(b)(c)(d)(f) 21 CFR 56.107 (a)(b)(c)(d) IRB-GB, (I)(B) FDA-IS, (FAQ)(II) FDA-IS, (CL)(VI) ICH-GCP, (3.2.1)	The IRB includes: 1.B.1. At least five members. 1.B.2. At least one member whose primary area of interest is non-scientific (e.g., lawyer, clergy, and ethicist). 1.B.3. At least one member whose primary area of interest is scientific. 1.B.4. At least one member who does not have any past or present association with the VA or university affiliate that would negate the status of a community, non-affiliated member. 1.B.5. Diversity of membership based on gender, cultural background, and sensitivity to community issues and/or community attitudes. 1.B.6. Members of more than one profession. 1.B.7. Affiliate IRBs have at least one member who is a VA representative. 1.B.8. Officials with responsibility for development and oversight of the HRPP are non-voting, ex-officio members.	Policies and procedures IRB membership lists, from the past year	Review of policies and procedures reflects compliance with regulations Review of IRB files shows compliance with requirements for current and past IRB members
1.C. The IRB meets regularly and with sufficient frequency, and members have sufficient time to review the materials prior to the meeting. Materials include the full protocol, a proposed informed consent form, any relevant	1.C.1. IRB meetings have the following arrangements: 1.C.1.1. The IRB has a set meeting schedule. 1.C.1.2. Except under specified "emergency" conditions, IRB members receive meeting materials	Policies and procedures IRB meeting schedule	Review of policies and procedures shows evidence of requirements Confirm existence of meeting schedule or regularly scheduled meeting date and time

merit review or grant applications, the investigator's brochure (if one exists), and any advertising intended to be seen or heard by potential subjects.	far enough in advance of the scheduled meeting to allow for sufficient review.	Distribution schedule IRB submission deadline schedule	(e.g., first Monday of the month at 8:00 a.m.)
	1.C.1.3. The IRB has established timelines for receipt by the IRB office and distribution of materials to members.	IRB member interview	Ask IRB member how soon before scheduled meetings they typically receive materials. Ask them whether they believe this is enough time to allow for sufficient review.
Regulation/Source 38 CFR 16.108(a)(1) 45 CFR 46.108(a)(1) 21 CFR 56.108(a)(1)	1.C.2. The IRB follows its established timelines.	IRB minutes	Review of IRB minutes for evidence of actual meeting dates conforming to scheduled dates
	1.C.3. The IRB periodically evaluates established timelines and it updates timelines to ensure effective participation of IRB members.	QI results	Review of QI results for evidence of compliance with meeting schedules
1.D. The IRB has a system for assigning reviewers to protocols prior to initial review (e.g., primary/secondary reviewer system), if applicable.	1.D.1. The IRB has a systematic process to assign review responsibility that is consistent with protocol content and reviewer expertise.	Policies and procedures	Review of policies and procedures for evidence of primary reviewer system, if applicable
	1.D.2. The IRB periodically evaluates the reviewer assignment system.	IRB member interview	IRB member is able to articulate the process for assigning protocols
Regulation/Source 38 CFR 16.107(a)		QI results	Review of QI results for evidence of compliance with, and appropriateness of, outlined protocol review system

IRB 2 The IRB systematically evaluates each research protocol to ensure adequate protection of human subjects in research.

Requirement	Element	Data Source	Method

2.A. There are written policies and procedures that describe IRB operations and functions.
 	
Regulation/Source
38 CFR 16.103(b)(4)(5)
38 CFR 16.108(a)(e)
38 CFR 6.115(a)(b)(6)
45 CFR 46.103(b)(4)(5)
45 CFR 46.115(a)(b)
21 CFR 56.108(a)(b)(c)
21 CFR 50.24
M-3, Part I, 9.09(c)(a)
IRB-GB, (I)(B)
FDA-IS, (CL)
ICH-GCP, (3.3)
MPA
VA Handbook
	2.A.1. These polices and procedures shall be consistent with all applicable VA and federal requirements and include the following:
	  2.A.1.1. Procedures and required information for conducting initial review and continuing review activities.
	    2.A.1.1.1. Procedures for reporting findings and actions to the investigator, the R&D Committee, and institutional officials as required.
	    2.A.1.1.2. Procedures for determining which projects require review more often than annually and which projects need verification from sources other than the investigators that no material changes have occurred since previous IRB review.
	  2.A.1.2. Procedures and criteria for making the following determinations for a research protocol: approval; require modifications in (to secure approval); or disapproval.
	  2.A.1.3. Procedures and criteria for suspension or termination of IRB approval of research protocols.
	  2.A.1.4. Criteria for when research protocols should include a Data Safety Monitoring Board (DSMB) as required by VA, DHHS, and FDA.
	  2.A.1.5. Review of protocol amendments, including procedures for determining crite-
		Policies and procedures	Review of policies and procedures shows evidence of requirements for IRB operations and functions

161

ria for what type of changes require full IRB review versus expedited review.
2.A.1.6. Procedures and criteria for determining if an expedited review process can be used.
2.A.1.7. Investigator reporting requirements, including:
  2.A.1.7.1. Providing IRB required data for continuing review.
  2.A.1.7.2. Submitting proposed changes in research protocol and/or consent forms for approval.
  2.A.1.7.3. Reporting deviations from approved protocol or other regulations and policies.
  2.A.1.7.4. Reporting adverse events.
  2.A.1.7.5. Reporting unanticipated problems involving risks to subjects.
  2.A.1.7.6. Submitting termination/completion reports.
2.A.1.8. Continuing review occurs at the specified time interval.			

2.B. The IRB reviews required and relevant information to make evaluations on research proposals during initial review.
 	
Regulation/Source
38 CFR 16.115(a)
45 CFR 46.115(a)
21 CFR 56.115(a)
FDA-IS, (FDA)(IV)
FDA-IS, (CL)(XI)
ICH-GCP, (3.1.2)(4.9.4)(8.0)
	2.B.1. The IRB considers the following at initial review:
	  2.B.1.1. Attestation, when required, by the investigator as to whether the proposal, or one substantially similar to it, has been disapproved by another IRB.
	  2.B.1.2. Scientific evaluations (if any) that accompany the proposal.
	  2.B.1.3. Research design.
	  2.B.1.4. Scientific rationale.
	  2.B.1.5. Statement of known and suspected risks and benefits.
		Initial review submission forms and checklists used by the IRB
		
		Sample of IRB initial review files
		
		IRB communications to investigators
			Review of submission form and checklists for requirements
			
			Review of protocols for evidence of content of requirements
			
			Review of IRB communications or other guidance for notice of submission requirements

OHRP-CFG
HHS-IGR

2.B.1.6. Procedures to minimize risks.
2.B.1.7. Recruitment and enrollment procedures, including payment to subjects.
2.B.1.8. Subject selection criteria.
2.B.1.9. Procedures to protect subject privacy and confidentiality.
2.B.1.10. Where appropriate, additional safeguards planned to protect the rights and welfare of potentially vulnerable subjects.
2.B.1.11. Process for monitoring and reporting adverse events.
2.B.1.12. Presence of a Data Safety Monitoring Board (DSMB) if applicable.
2.B.1.13. Other information to be used for recruitment or to inform subjects or potential subjects about the nature of the research.
2.B.1.14. Scientific training and qualifications of investigator and research staff.
2.B.1.15. Human subject protection training of investigators and research staff.
2.B.1.16. Investigator potential financial conflicts.
2.B.1.17. Proposed informed consent documents.
2.B.2. Based on its review of the information above, the IRB approves, requires modifications, or disapproves proposed research.
2.B.3. The IRB conducts audits of the adequacy of information at initial review. Results are used for QI purposes and actions taken, as needed.

IRB minutes

QI results

Review of IRB minutes shows IRB consideration of requirements as appropriate, and decisions to approve are not pro forma

Review of QI results shows evidence of assessment of requirements for initial submission

2.C. The IRB uses required and relevant information to conduct continuing review of research proposals and makes recommended changes. *Regulation/Source* 38 CFR 16.1.09 (e) M-3, Part 1, 9.09 (f) 45 CFR 46 1.09 (e) 21 CFR 56 1.09 (f)	2.C.1. In addition to copies of the documents required for the initial review, the IRB considers the following information, where applicable, for continuing review: 2.C.1.1. Currently approved informed consent documents.	Policy and procedures	Review of policies and procedures shows evidence of requirements for submission of continuing review
	2.C.1.2. Approved or proposed amendments, including minor changes (if any), and the IRB action on each amendment.	Continuing review submission forms	Forms have requirements listed
	2.C.1.3. Research findings to date. 2.C.1.4. Reports of injuries to subjects. 2.C.1.5. All serious adverse events or unanticipated problems involving risks to subjects.	Checklists and forms used by IRB	IRB checklists show evidence of IRB consideration of required information
	2.C.1.6. Recent published medical or scientific studies applicable to the protocol. 2.C.1.7. Review of information that may change risk/benefit ratio, including adverse events or unanticipated problems. 2.C.1.8. Documentation of protocol violations and/or deviations. 2.C.1.9. Documentation of non-compliance with applicable regulations.	Sample of IRB continuing review files	Protocols reviewed show evidence of IRB consideration of required information and that continuing review was submitted and considered within the required time frame for the protocol
	2.C.1.10. Number of subjects enrolled and entered into the study. 2.C.1.10.1. Gender and minority status of subjects entered into the protocol.	IRB communications to investigators	IRB communications list requirements for continuing review submission
	2.C.1.10.2. Number of subjects in each of the following categories: children, prisoners, pregnant women, economically disadvantaged, decisionally impaired, or homeless. 2.C.1.11. Number of subjects withdrawn by self and by investigator, and reasons for withdrawal. 2.C.1.12. Review of a summary of the	IRB minutes	IRB minutes reflect consideration of requirements

DSMB meetings (if applicable) or findings based on information collected on AEs, UAEs, and SAEs as required by the approved data and safety monitoring plan.

2.C.1.12.1. An assurance that all SAEs and UAEs have been reported as required.

2.C.1.12.2. Review of IND/IDE safety reports and MedWatch reports.

2.C.1.13. Any new recruitment documents.

2.C.2. Based on its review of the above information, the IRB decides that the research can be continued, continued with modifications, suspended, or terminated.

2.C.3. Based on its continuing review, the IRB requires appropriate changes to the following:

2.C.3.1. Informed consent form content.

2.C.3.2. Frequency of continuing review.

2.C.3.3. Level of safety monitoring.

2.C.4. The IRB conducts audits of the adequacy of information considered at continuing review.

2.C.4.1. Results are used for QI purposes and actions taken, as needed.

2.D. The IRB has policies and procedures for the conduct of expedited review (if applicable) and appropriately utilizes such review.

Regulation/Source
38 CFR 16.110
M-3, Part I, 9.10
45 CFR 46.110
21 CFR 56.110

2.D.1. The IRB's policies and procedures for expedited review conform to VA and federal regulations and include:

2.D.1.1 The IRB identifies categories of research for which expedited review is allowed.

2.D.1.2. There are established qualifications and experience criteria for those IRB members who serve as chairperson's designee(s) in conducting expedited review.

2.D.1.3. The IRB must have criteria for establishing that research involves no more

Policies and procedures	Review of policies and procedures for evidence of requirements for expedited review
IRB submission forms and checklists used by the IRB	Review of IRB submission forms for requirements for expedited review
Sample of IRB expedited review files	Review of protocols approved through expedited

FDA-IS, (FAQ)(20)
FDA-IS, (CL)(IX)(C)
OHRP-CFG (B)

than minimal risk.

2.D.1.4. The IRB must have criteria for establishing that changes in previously approved research are "minor."

2.D.1.5. The IRB has methods to keep IRB members advised of research proposals approved under expedited review that include documentation of specific permissible categories justifying expedited review.

2.D.2. The IRB conducts expedited review of protocols in conformance with its policies and procedures.

2.D.2.1. Expedited review shall be conducted by IRB Chairperson or by one or more experienced IRB members designated by the IRB Chairperson.

2.D.2.2. Expedited reviews comply with the IRB policies and procedures and applicable VA and federal regulations.

2.D.3. The IRB conducts audits or self-assessments of compliance with VA and federal regulations and its policies and procedures on expedited review.

2.D.3.1. Results are used for QI purposes and actions taken, as needed.

IRB minutes

review shows that the protocols met criteria

IRB minutes show that protocols reviewed through expedited review were presented to full committee for consideration

Standard	Detail	Evidence	Review Criteria
2.E. The IRB has policies and procedures for determining whether research involving human subjects is exempt from IRB review and correctly makes such determinations. *Regulation/Source* 38 CFR 16.101(b) M-3, Part I, 9.06 45 CFR 46.101(b) IRB-GB, (I)(A)	2.E.1. The IRB policies and procedures for determining exempt status conform to VA and federal regulations and include: 2.E.1.1. Definition of all categories of research that are exempt from IRB review. 2.E.1.2. Process for determining exempt status. 2.E.2. The IRB makes determination of exempt status in accordance with federal regulations. 2.E.3. The IRB conducts audits or self-assessments of compliance with VA and federal regulations and its policies and procedures on exempt status. 2.E.3.1. Results are used for QI and actions taken, as needed.	Policies and procedures IRB minutes IRB Chair interview IRB coordinator interview QI results	Review of policies and procedures for presence of requirements for exempt status IRB minutes show evidence of evaluation of protocols for exempt status. IRB Chair is able to discuss application of exempt status at the institution IRB coordinator is able to discuss process for determining exempt status QI results show evidence of compliance with VA and federal regulations and IRB policies and procedures on the determination of exempt status
2.F. The IRB has policies and procedures for determination of risk level of investigational devices, appropriately makes such determinations, and implements any resulting actions. *Regulation/Source* 21 CFR 812.62, 66 FDA-IS, (SR/NSR)	2.F.1. The IRB's policies and procedures for the review of investigational devices address the following: 2.F.1.1. The IRB decision is based on proposed use of the device and not the device alone. 2.F.1.2. The IRB may agree or disagree with the sponsor's assessment of significant risk or nonsignificant risk. 2.F.1.3. The IRB notifies the sponsor and investigator when it determines the device is	Policies and procedures IRB minutes Sample of device protocols	Review of policies and procedures for determination of risk level of devices IRB minutes reflect evaluation of risk level of device Review of device protocols contains evidence of risk level of device

a significant risk device and proceeds to review the study only after an IDE is obtained by the sponsor.

2.F.1.4. The IRB proceeds to review the study under requisite criteria for any study when the device is determined to be non-significant risk.

2.F.2. The IRB conducts audits or self-assessments of compliance with VA and federal regulations for assessing whether the investigational devices are significant or non-significant risk.

2.F.2.1. Results are used for QI and actions taken, as needed.

QI results

QI results show evidence of compliance with VA and federal regulations and IRB policies and procedures on the determination of risk level of devices

IRB 3 The IRB maintains documentation of its activities.

Requirement	Element	Data Source	Method

3.A. The IRB documents discussions and decisions on research proposals and activities.
 	
Regulation/Source
38 CFR 16.115(a)(2)
M-3, Part 1,
9.09(g)(1)(b)
45 CFR 46.115(a)(2)
21 CFR 56.115(a)(2)
IRB-GB, (I)(B)
FDA-IS, (CL)(X)
ICH-GCP, (3.4)
OHRP-CFG (G64)
	3.A.1. Minutes of IRB meetings contain sufficient detail to show:
	3.A.1.1. Attendance.
	3.A.1.2. Approval of previous meeting minutes.
	3.A.1.3. Actions taken by the IRB at the meeting.
	3.A.1.4. The vote on actions, including the number of members voting for, against, and abstaining.
	   3.A.1.4.1. Names of members abstaining.
	   3.A.1.4.2. Quorum requirements were met at each recorded vote or for the entire meeting, including circumstances in which members recused themselves due to conflicts of interest.
	   3.A.1.4.3. A non-scientific member of the IRB was present during the entire meeting.
	3.A.2. When an IRB member has a real or potential conflict of interest relative to the proposal under consideration, the minutes will document that the IRB member did not participate in the deliberations or voting on the proposal and that the quorum was maintained.
	3.A.3. Minutes document the basis for requiring changes in or disapproving research and documentation of resolution of these
		Policies and procedures
		
		IRB minutes
		
		IRB communications
		
		R&D Committee minutes
			Review of policies and procedures shows evidence of evaluation of requirements for content of IRB minutes
			
			IRB minutes contain required information
			
			IRB communications to investigators, R&D Committee, or other institutional officials document decisions made by the IRB
			
			R&D Committee minutes document acknowledgement of IRB decisions

issues when resolution occurs.

3.A.4. Minutes document required IRB findings where needed to approve exceptions, waivers, or use of vulnerable populations.

3.A.5. Minutes include a written summary of the discussion of:

    3.A.5.1. Controverted issues and their resolution.

    3.A.5.2. Risk/benefit analysis.

    3.A.5.3. Informed consent.

    3.A.5.4. Risk level of investigational devices.

    3.A.5.5. Additional safeguards to protect vulnerable populations if entered as study subjects.

3.A.6. Minutes reflect results of expedited reviews and the eligibility category serving as justification for meeting expedited review criteria.

3.A.7. Minutes include items approved as exempt from review and documentation of the eligibility category serving as justification for the exemption.

3.A.8. Minutes document the frequency of continuing review of each research project, based upon the degree of risk, as determined by the IRB.

3.A.9. IRB decisions are reported promptly and in writing to the investigator and appropriate institutional officials. In addition, suspensions and terminations are reported to the department or agency head.

3.A.10. IRB minutes are completed in a timely manner and forwarded to the R&D Committee.

3.B. The IRB retains required records for at least 3 years from study completion. *Regulation/Source* 38 CFR 16.115(b) M-3, Part 1, 9.09(g)(2) 45 CFR 46.115(b) 21 CFR 56.115(b) IRB-GB, (I)(B) FDA-IS, (CL)(X)(I) ICH-GCP (3.4)	3.B.1. Required records are retained for a minimum of 3 years following the completion of the study, in accordance with VHA's Records Control Schedule, applicable FDA and DHHS regulations, or as required by sponsors.	Policies and procedures	Review of policies and procedures shows evidence of requirements for record retention and access
	3.B.2. All records shall be accessible for inspection and copying by authorized representatives of VA, including accreditors and appropriate federal departments or agencies, at reasonable times and in a reasonable manner.	IRB files	IRB files are kept in a secure location
	3.B.3. IRB records are the property and the responsibility of the local research office and are maintained and/or stored as required to protect the privacy and confidentiality of subjects. Records must be stored in a secure environment (e.g., locking file cabinets).	IRB coordinator interview	Staff demonstrates filing system to show that files are kept in an organized fashion in a secure location
	3.B.4. There must be limited access to the files.	IRB file access log	Review of access log reflects access by appropriate individuals or groups
	3.B.4.1. There must be logs or records of access to restricted files, including: 3.B.4.1.1. Who accessed the files, with the exception of IRB and research office staff; 3.B.4.1.2. What files were accessed; 3.B.4.1.3. When the files were accessed; 3.B.4.1.4. For what purpose the files were accessed.		Additionally, all research proposals and IRB minutes requested for the survey process were available.

TABLE C-4 CONSIDERATIONS OF RISKS AND BENEFITS

Rationale

All research should be designed to maximize possible benefits and minimize possible harms to participants. When a research proposal does not have the proper balance of risks and benefits, it should not be approved. One of the major responsibilities of the IRB is to assess the risks and benefits of the proposed research and to put in place safeguards that require investigators to act in ways that minimize harms to subjects. This standard contains the requirements for IRB actions related to assessment and balancing of risks and benefits.

KEY:

CFR = Code of Federal Regulations
M-3, Part 1 = The Veterans Affairs Manual, Chapter 9
IRB-GB = OPRR IRB Guidebook
FDA-IS = FDA Information Sheets
FDA-IS, (CL) = Appendix H: A Self-Evaluation Checklist for IRBs
FDA-IS, (FAQ) = Frequently Asked Question
FDA-IS, (ICG) = The Guide to Informed Consent
FDA-IS, (CR) = Continuing Review After Study Approval
ICH-GCP = International Conference on Harmonization, Good Clinical Practice Guideline
OHRP-CFG = Office of Human Research Protections Compliance Activities: Common Findings and Guidance 9/1/2000

RB 1 The IRB systematically evaluates risks and anticipated benefits as part of the initial review and ongoing review of research.

Requirement	Element	Data Source	Method

1.A. The IRB has procedures (e.g., evaluation tools to be completed by reviewers) for initial review of the risks and benefits of research.
 	
Regulation/Source
38 CFR 16.111(a)(1)(2)
M-3, Part 1, 9.09(a)(1)
45 CFR 46.103(b)(4)
45 CFR 46.111(a)(1)(2)
21CFR 56.111(a)(1)(2)
IRB-GB, (III)(A)
	1.A.1. Procedures for the initial review of the risks and benefits of research include:
	  1.A.1.1. Identification of the risks associated with research.
	  1.A.1.2. Assessment of whether risks have been minimized.
	  1.A.1.3. Determination of the level of risk of the research (e.g., minimal, greater than minimal).
	1.A.1.4. Identification of the probable individual and societal benefits of the research.
	1.A.1.5. Determination that risks are reasonable in relation to the benefits to subjects and the knowledge to be gained.
	1.A.1.6. Determination of intervals for continuing review based on the level of risk.
		Procedures for the evaluation of risks and benefits
		
		IRB member interview
			Review of procedures for the presence of each element
			
			IRB member describes processes for the evaluation of risks associated with research proposals

1.B. The IRB consistently identifies and analyzes potential sources of risk and the measures to minimize risk. *Regulation/Source* 38 CFR 16.111(a)(1)(2) M-3, Part 1, 9.09(a)(1)(a) 45 CFR 46.111(a)(1)(2) 21 CFR 56.111(a)(1)(2) IRB-GB, (III)(A)	1.B.1. The IRB's evaluation of research proposal risk includes consideration of the following: 1.B.1.1. Research design. 1.B.1.2. Scientific rationale. 1.B.1.3. Research plan for the frequency of monitoring of the data collected to ensure the safety of subjects. 1.B.1.4. Training and competence of investigator and research staff. 1.B.1.5. Category of vulnerability of the proposed study population, where applicable. 1.B.2. The IRB distinguishes the risks of research activities from the risk of therapeutic activities. 1.B.3. The IRB ensures that the proposed research minimizes risk through the following: 1.B.3.1. Uses sound research design which does not unnecessarily expose subjects to risk. 1.B.3.2. Uses diagnostic or treatment modalities already being performed on the subjects. 1.B.4. The IRB identifies physical, psychological, social, and economic risks, including risks to privacy and the probability of occurrence posed by research design, interventions, and procedures. 1.B.5. When reviewing a research proposal with elements warranting special attention (e.g., placebos, challenge studies, radiation exposure, deviations from standards of care), the IRB specifically considers the appropriateness of, and rationale for, such elements and documents such consideration.	IRB minutes Sample of reviewed protocols, protocol evaluation tools, and IRB minutes IRB member interview QI reports	Review of IRB minutes shows that each research proposal has been evaluated for the elements of the standard Review of protocols for evidence that the IRB identified and evaluated all sources of risk in 1.B.4. and probability of risk Ask IRB member to describe how IRB evaluates sources of risk and measure to minimize risk Review QI reports for evidence of compliance in evaluating and documenting sources of risk and measures to minimize risk

Requirement	Element	Data Source	Method
1.C. The IRB evaluates each research proposal to identify the probable benefits of the research. *Regulation/Source* 38 CFR 16.111(a)(1)(2) M-3, Part 1, 9.09(a)(2)(a) 45 CFR 46.111(a)(1)(2) 21 CFR 6.111(a)(1)(2) IRB-GB, (III)(A)	1.C.1. The IRB identifies the limit of anticipated benefits research subjects may derive from participation in the research. 1.C.2. The IRB determines the importance of the knowledge that may be reasonably expected to result from the research. (The IRB should consider only the specific risks and benefits that may result from the research.)	IRB minutes IRB evaluation tools (or checklists) IRB member interview QI reports	Review of IRB minutes or completed protocol evaluation tools document assessment of anticipated benefits IRB members identify methods for determining anticipated benefits of research proposals Review QI reports for evidence of IRB compliance with procedures for assessing anticipated benefits of research proposals

RB 1 The IRB systematically evaluates risks and anticipated benefits as part of the initial review and ongoing review of research.

Requirement	Element	Data Source	Method
1.D. The IRB determines that risks to subjects are reasonable in relation to anticipated benefits. *Regulation/Source* 38 CFR 16.111(a)(1)(2) M-3, Part 1, 9.09(a)(2)(a) 45 CFR 46.111(a)(1)(2) 21 CFR 56.111(a)(1)(2) IRB-GB, (III)(A)	1.D.1. The IRB determines the risks to subjects are reasonable in relation to anticipated benefits, if any, to subjects, and the importance of the knowledge that may be expected to result.	IRB minutes IRB evaluation tools (or checklists) IRB member interview QI reports	Review of IRB minutes or completed protocol evaluation tools document assessment of risk/benefit ratio IRB members identify methods for determining risk/benefit ratio of research proposals Review QI reports for evidence of IRB compliance with procedures for assessing risk/benefit ratio of research proposals
1.E. The IRB continually evaluates the risks and benefits of ongoing proto-	1.E.1. The IRB determines for each approved research protocol, the specific interval for periodic review of risks and determines the need	IRB minutes	Minutes show review and discussion about whether there is a change in risk or action required

cols.

Regulation/Source	Criteria		
	for monitoring safety. 1.E.2. The IRB demonstrates ongoing review of the following sources of risks and benefits:		
38 CFR 16.109(e) 38 CFR 16.111(a)(6) M-3, Part 1, 9.09(f) 45 CFR 46.109(e)	1.E.2.1 Evaluation of adverse event reports from investigators. 1.E.2.2. Evaluation of sponsor safety reports (e.g., IND or IDE).	IRB communications	Communications to investigators document decision about changes in risk or actions required
45 CFR 46.111(a)(6) 21 CFR 56.109(f) 21 CFR 56.111(a)(6)	1.E.2.3. Evaluation of MedWatch reports. 1.E.2.4. Evaluation of amended or updated Investigator Brochures.	Completed IRB continuing review tools	Sample of approved protocol files show documentation of consideration of risks and benefits at continuing reviews
	1.E.2.5. Evaluation of amendments to protocols. 1.E.2.6. Evaluation of any new information available regarding the research project.	IRB serious adverse event reporting forms, safety reports, MedWatch reports	Sample of approved protocol files show documentation of consideration of risks and benefits at review of SAE, safety reports, and MedWatch reports

TABLE C-5 RECRUITMENT AND SUBJECT SELECTION

Rationale

Because research frequently poses risks of harm and the possibility of benefit, it is necessary to fairly distribute potential risks and benefits. It is also necessary to protect groups that have been discriminated against in the past, who are vulnerable to manipulation, or unable to freely consent, from the risks of research. IRBs must assure that procedures for selecting research subjects are fair. This standard outlines the expected processes that IRBs must use to ensure that research participants are identified and recruited properly.

KEY:

CFR = Code of Federal Regulations
M-3, Part 1 = The Veterans Affairs Manual, Chapter 9
IRB-GB = OPRR IRB Guidebook
FDA-IS = FDA Information Sheets
FDA-IS, (CL) = Appendix H: A Self-Evaluation Checklist for IRBs
FDA-IS, (FAQ) = Frequently Asked Questions
FDA-IS, (ICG) = The Guide to Informed Consent
FDA-IS, (CR) = Continuing Review After Study Approval
FDA-IS, (RSS) = Recruiting Study Subjects
FDA-IS, (PRS) = Payment to Research Subjects
ICH-GCP = International Conference on Harmonization, Good Clinical Practice Guidelines
HHS IGR = HHS Inspector General's Report

RSS 1 The IRB systematically evaluates recruitment and subject selection practices.

Requirement	Element	Data Source	Method
1.A. The IRB defines acceptable recruitment practices for proposed research. *Regulation/Source* HHS-IGR M-3 Part I, 9.13 FDA-IS, (RSS) FDA-IS, (PRS)	The IRB's policies and procedures define acceptable recruitment practices as applied to the following: 1.A.1. Payment to subjects. 1.A.2. Advertisements. 1.A.3. Compensation to investigators, physicians, and other health care providers for identifying and/or enrolling subjects.	Policies and procedures	Review of policies and procedures for the presence of each element of the requirement
1.B. The IRB reviews subject recruitment methods, advertising materials, and subject payment arrangements proposed, and determines that they are fair and appropriate. *Regulation/Source* HHS-IGR M-3 Part I, 9.13 FDA-IS, (RSS) FDA-IS, (PRS)	The IRB demonstrates that it has considered the following recruitment practices as part of its review: 1.B.1. The nature or amount of the compensation offered to subjects for participation in research does not create undue influence, particularly for economically disadvantaged subjects. 1.B.2. Claims made in advertisements appropriately reflect the study protocol.	IRB minutes	IRB minutes document discussion of recruitment practices for protocols
		Completed IRB protocol evaluation tools	Completed evaluation tools demonstrate evaluation of recruitment practices
		Sample of reviewed protocol advertisements (both approved and disapproved)	Approved advertisements contain appropriate information and are consistent with protocol content
		Sample of protocols for subject information materials	Approved subject information materials contain appropriate information and are consistent with protocol content

Criterion/Standard	Regulation/Source	Source of Evidence	Verification Method
1.C. The IRB has policies and procedures to evaluate the equitable selection of subjects in proposed research and considers subject selection in its review of research. The IRB has policies and procedures for and implements the following: 1.C.1. Purposes of research. 1.C.2. Setting in which research occurs. 1.C.3. Plan for soliciting subjects. 1.C.4. The scientific and ethical justification for including vulnerable populations such as children, prisoners, pregnant women, mentally disabled persons, or economically or educationally disadvantaged persons (e.g., the homeless).	*Regulation/Source* 38 CFR 16.111(a)(3) M-3 Part I, 9.09 (a)(3) 45 CFR 46.111(a)(3) 21 CFR 56.111(a)(3) IRB-GB, (III)(C)	Policies and procedures	Review of policies and procedures for the presence of required elements
		IRB application forms	Review of IRB application for evidence of collection of recruitment plans
1.D. The IRB determines that proposed subject selection (inclusion and exclusion criteria and recruitment procedures) is equitable with respect to the distribution of the burdens and benefits of the proposed research. The IRB considers the following criteria: 1.D.1. The purpose of the research requires or justifies using the proposed subject population. 1.D.2. The burdens and benefits of research are fairly distributed. 1.D.3. Where specific populations are over- or under-represented in the proposed subject population, the rationale for such over- or under-representation is justified. 1.D.4. Subject selection is consistent with VA and HHS policies on the participation of women, children, and minorities in medical research involving human subjects.		IRB minutes	IRB minutes show evidence of IRB consideration of equitable selection
		Sample of reviewed research proposals.	Protocols show evidence of subject selection considerations
			Protocols show evidence consideration of VA and HHS policies on participation of women, children, and minorities

1.D.5. *When the causes or risk of the research*

38 CFR
16.111(a)(3)
M-3 Part I, 9.09
(a)(3)
45 CFR
46.111(a)(3)
21 CFR
56.111(a)(3)
IRB-GB, (III)(C)
HHS IGR

justifies the inclusion of vulnerable populations as subjects (e.g., children, prisoners, pregnant women, mentally disabled persons, or economically or educationally disadvantaged persons), the IRB determines that additional safeguards have been included in the study to protect the rights and welfare of these subjects and specifically documents those safeguards.

Protocols show evidence of additional safeguards for subject selection in vulnerable populations

TABLE C-6 PRIVACY AND CONFIDENTIALITY

Rationale

Violation of a research subject's privacy may lead to significant harm from loss of work, embarrassment, loss of benefits, and loss of dignity. IRBs must ensure that proposed research protects human subjects from loss of privacy and breach of confidentiality. This requires that IRBs understand the risks of harm from loss of confidentiality, and methods, such as de-identifying data, that may reduce the risk of breach of confidentiality. This standard outlines requirements for the protection of privacy and confidentiality.

KEY:

CFR = Code of Federal Regulations
M-3, Part 1 = The Veterans Affairs Manual, Chapter 9
IRB-GB = OPRR IRB Guidebook
FDA-IS = FDA Information Sheets
FDA-IS, (CL) = Appendix H: A Self-Evaluation Checklist for IRBs
FDA-IS, (FAQ) = Frequently Asked Questions
FDA-IS, (ICG) = The Guide to Informed Consent
FDA-IS, (CR) = Continuing Review After Study Approval
ICH-GCP = International Conference on Harmonization, Good Clinical Practice Guideline

PC 1 The IRB systematically evaluates the protection of privacy and confidentiality in proposed research.

Requirement	Element	Data Source	Method
1.A. The IRB has policies and procedures to evaluate provisions for the protection of privacy and confidentiality which conform to VA, federal, and local requirements. *Regulation/Source* 38 CFR 16.111(a)(7) 38 CFR 17.33(a)(1) 38 CFR 17.33(b)(1)(v) 38 CFR 17.33(f) M-3, Part I, 909 (a)(7) 45 CFR 46.111(a)(7) 21 CFR 56.111(a)(7) IRB-GB, (III)(D)	The IRB has policies and procedures which set forth, for investigators, the requirements for preserving privacy and confidentiality. Consideration must be given to: 1.A.1. Methods used to obtain information about participants and potential participants. 1.A.2. Nature of information being sought. 1.A.3. Use of personally identifiable records. 1.A.4. Plan to protect the confidentiality of research data that may include coding, removal of identifying information, limiting access to data, use of Certificates of Confidentiality, or other effective methods. 1.A.5. The investigator's disclosures to participants about confidentiality. 1.A.6. Determination of whether a federal Certificate of Confidentiality should be obtained.	Policy and procedures Guidance to investigators	Review of policies and procedures for the presence of each element Guidance materials provided to investigators contain specifications for disclosure to participants in consent forms or other patient information
1.B. The IRB systematically assesses research proposals for provisions to protect privacy and confidentiality.	1.B.1. The IRB evaluates the following: 1.B.1.1. Methods used to	Sample of completed IRB protocol evaluation forms or IRB minutes	IRB evaluation forms or minutes demonstrate assessment of privacy and confidentiality issues associ-

Regulation/Source			
38 CFR 16.111(a)(7) 38 CFR 17.33(a)(1) 38 CFR 17.33(b)(1)(v) 38 CFR 17.33(f) M-3, Part I, 909 (a)(7) 45 CFR 46.111(a)(7) 21 CFR 56.111(a)(7) IRB-GB, (III)(D)	identify and recruit participants protect patient privacy and confidentiality. 1.B.1.2. Methods to obtain information about participants are reasonable and protect privacy. 1.B.1.3. There are adequate provisions for protecting the confidentiality of research data, including, where appropriate, Certificates of Confidentiality. 1.B.1.4. The informed consent form and other information presented to potential research participants adequately discloses the risks to privacy and confidentiality. 1.B.2. The IRB conducts audits or self-assessments of compliance with privacy and confidentiality requirements. 1.B.2.1. Results of audits or self-assessments are used for QI and actions are taken, as needed.	IRB application forms QI reports	ated with the protocol Review of IRB application for presence of each element Review of QI reports for evidence of compliance with policies and procedures

TABLE C-7 INFORMED CONSENT

Rationale

Informed consent is critical to the protection of human research subjects. It permits participants to determine whether they are willing to accept the risks of the research in order to gain the potential benefits. Requirements for informed consent are met when potential participants are: 1) capable of deciding whether to participate; 2) adequately informed about the risks and benefits of participation; 3) able to understand the information; and 4) voluntarily decide to participate. This standard outlines the requirements for processes that research programs and IRBs must follow in assessing whether informed consent is adequate.

KEY:

CFR = Code of Federal Regulations
M-3, Part 1 = The Veterans Affairs Manual, Chapter 9
IRB-GB = OPRR IRB Guidebook
FDA-IS = FDA Information Sheets
FDA-IS, (CL) = Appendix H: A Self-Evaluation Checklist for IRBs
FDA-IS, (FAQ) = Frequently Asked Questions
FDA-IS, (ICG) = The Guide to Informed Consent
FDA-IS, (CR) = Continuing Review After Study Approval
FDA-IS, (PRS) = Payment to Research Subjects
ICH-GCP = International Conference on Harmonization, Good Clinical Practice Guideline NBAC = National Bioethics Advisory Commission Report

IC 1 The IRB assures that prospective human subjects give valid informed consent.

Requirement	Element	Data Source	Method

1.A. The IRB has policies and procedures for the process of obtaining informed consent from subjects or their legally authorized representatives and ensures compliance with policies and procedures.
 	
Regulation/Source
38 CFR 16.116
38 CFR 16.111(a)(4)
M-3, Part 1, 9.09(a)(4)
45 CFR 46.111(a)(4)
45 CFR 46.116
21 CFR 50.20
21 CFR 50.25
ICH-GCP 4.8.5
FDA-IS, (ICG)
	1.A.1. IRB policies and procedures describe the following:
	  1.A.1.1. The IRB has the authority to observe the consent process.
	  1.A.1.2. Who, under VA policy, state, and local law, may serve as a legally authorized representative for subjects determined to be incapable of making an autonomous decision. (There is a distinction between treatment authorization and research authorization).
	  1.A.1.3. Who is eligible to inform the prospective subject about all aspects of the trial and conduct the informed consent process.
	  1.A.1.4. Consent is obtained prior to the conduct of any procedures required by the protocol.
	1.A.2. In its review of research proposals, the IRB ensures that the investigative staff conducts the informed consent process with the following considerations:
	  1.A.2.1 Assessing the subject's capacity to consent to a research protocol.
	  1.A.2.2. Ensuring that information is given to the subject, or his or her legally authorized representative in
		Policies and procedures for the process of obtaining consent
		
		IRB communications to investigators regarding the consent process including Investigator Handbooks/Guidelines
		
		IRB documentation of observation of consent process
		
		IRB minutes
		
		QI results
			Review of policies and procedures for evidence of elements of consent process
			
			Review of IRB communications for instructions to investigators on the IRB's requirements for the consent process
			
			Review of IRB documentation of consent process observations shows critical evaluation of the process with recommendations for improvement
			
			Review of IRB minutes for evidence of consideration of proposed consent processes
			
			QI results show evidence of investigator compliance with consent process guidelines

Standard	Documentation	Verification
language that is understandable to the subject or representative. 1.A.2.3. Providing the prospective subject or the legally authorized representative sufficient opportunity to consider whether or not to participate. 1.A.2.4. Ensuring that subjects give consent without coercion or undue influence. 1.A.3. The IRB conducts audits or self-assessments to assess investigator compliance with regulatory requirements. 1.A.3.1 The IRB uses the results for QI purposes and takes action, as needed.		
1.B. The IRB has policies and procedures that define the required content for informed consent forms and ensures compliance with these policies and procedures. *Regulation/Source* 38 CFR 16.116 M-3, Part 1, 9.09(4)(5) and Appendix 9C Procedures for Obtaining Informed Consent 45 CFR 46.116 21 CFR 50.20-27 FDA-IS, (FAQ)(V)(VI) IRB-GB, (III)(B) FDA-IS, (PRS) 1.B.1. The IRB requires that consent forms include all the basic elements of information as set forth in VA and other federal regulations. 1.B.2. The IRB requires the consent form to contain information in language understandable to the subject or the representative. 1.B.2.1. Based on the potential population, the appropriate reading level of consent forms is defined. 1.B.2.2. Validated translations of consent forms are required for non-English-speaking subjects. 1.B.3. The IRB identifies those circumstances when the investigator must provide any of the additional	Policies and procedures outlining consent content requirements IRB template consent Sample of IRB-approved consent forms IRB minutes documenting consent analysis QI results	Review of Policies and Procedures for consistency with regulations and all elements of the requirement Review of IRB template consent for consistency with regulations (Checklist contains all 8 required elements) Review of sample of IRB-approved consent forms for evidence of consistency with regulations Review of IRB minutes for evidence of evaluation, documentation of requested changes to consent forms to comply with regulations, and investigator compliance.

elements of information as set forth in VA and other Federal regulations.

1.B.4. The IRB requires all information concerning payment to subjects, including the amount and schedule of payments, to be included in the informed consent document.

1.B.5. The IRB requires the content of consent forms to be consistent with state laws regarding content (if applicable).

1.B.6. The IRB prohibits any informed consent, whether oral or written, from including any exculpatory language through which the subject or the legally authorized representative is made to waive or appear to waive any of the subject's legal rights, or releases or appears to release the investigator, the sponsor, the institution, or its agents from liability for negligence.

1.B.7. The IRB conducts audits or self-assessments to determine that only approved consent forms are used and have the required content.

1.B.7.1. The IRB uses the results for QI purposes and takes action, as needed.

QI results show evidence of compliance in evaluating consents for VA, federal, local, and institutional requirements and that only approved consent forms are used by investigative staff.

1.C. The IRB has policies and procedures regarding documentation of informed consent and ensures that investigators and staff conform to these policies and procedures

1.C.1. The IRB requires informed consent to be documented by the use of a written consent form, VA Form 10-1086, approved by the IRB and signed by the subject or the subject's legally authorized representative

Policies and procedures for documentation of informed consent

Review of policies and procedures for evidence of requirements for consent documentation

IRB template consent

Review of template consent for required signature and date lines

Regulation/Source			
38 CFR 16.117(c) M-3, Part 1, 9.11 45 CFR 46.117(c) 21 CFR 50.23(a) 21 CFR 50.27(b)(2) IRB-GB, (III)(B)	1.C.1.1. Consent forms contain the required signature lines. 1.C.1.1.1. Subject signature and date of signature.	Sample of approved consents	Review of sample of IRB-approved consents for evidence of required signature lines
	1.C.1.1.2. Signature of person conducting the informed consent process.	IRB minutes	Review of IRB minutes for documentation of evaluation for use of short-form consent
	1.C.1.1.3. Witness to the signature. 1.C.1.1.4. Investigator, if an investigator did not conduct the consent process.	Sample of protocols where short-form consent is used	Review of sample of protocols with short-form consents for evidence of requirements for appropriateness of use
	1.C.1.1.5. Witness signature on "short form."	IRB communications	Review of communications to investigators regarding the requirements for documentation of consent
	1.C.2. Policies describe situations where the signature of a witness is required. 1.C.3. Policies describe conditions under which a "short form" informed consent may be used.	Sample of signed consent forms QI results	Review of sample of signed consent forms for presence of required signatures
	1.C.4. The IRB conducts audits to determine that investigators have documented informed consent through the use of the approved consent form, dated and signed, with a copy given to the subject or legally authorized representative, and the original is kept in the medical record.		Review of QI results for evidence of IRB evaluation of consents and compliance of investigators with requirements for documentation of consent.
	1.C.4.1. In conjunction with the use of an IRB-approved "short form," the IRB-approved written summary of what was said to the subject or legally authorized representative, is signed by the witness. 1.C.4.2. The IRB uses the results		

Standard	Evidence	Method of review
1.D. The IRB has policies and procedures for approving waiver or alteration of the informed consent form and complies with these policies and procedures. *Regulation/Source* 38 CFR 16.116 38 CFR 16.117 M-3, part 1, 9.11 45 CFR 46.116 45 CFR 46.117 21 CFR 50.109(c) IRB-GB, (III)(B) FDA-IS, (ICG)		
for QI purposes and takes action, as needed. 1.D.1. The IRB defines the conditions under which it will permit waiver or alteration of any element of informed consent to include: 1.D.1.1. The research involves no more than minimal risk. 1.D.1.2. The waiver or alteration will not adversely affect the rights of the subjects. 1.D.1.3. The research could not be practically done without such waiver or alteration. 1.D.1.4. Whenever appropriate, the subjects will be provided with additional pertinent information after participation. 1.D.1.5. The research or demonstration project is to be conducted by, or subject to the approval of, state or local government officials and is designed to study, evaluate, or otherwise examine public benefit of service programs, procedures for obtaining benefits or services under those programs, possible changes in or alternatives to those programs, or possible changes in methods or levels of payment for benefits or services under those programs. 1.D.2. The IRB does not allow waiver or alteration of informed consent	Policies and procedures for waiving or altering consent	Review of policies and procedures for conditions for waiving or altering consent, content
	Sample of protocols	Review of protocols where consent was waived or altered for assurance that conditions were met
	IRB minutes	IRB minutes show evidence of evaluation of conditions for waiver or alterations of consent content consistent with policies and procedures
	QI results	QI results show evaluation of and compliance with conditions for waiving or altering consent, content

forms when FDA-regulated test articles are involved.

1.D.3. In its approval of waiver or alteration, the IRB documents its specific findings that conditions permitting waiver or alteration are met.

1.D.4. In its decision to waive the requirement for the investigator to obtain a signed informed consent form for some or all subjects, the IRB documents the regulatory basis for such waiver, providing either that:

1.D.4.1. The only record linking the subject and the research would be the consent document and the principal risk would be potential harm resulting from breach of confidentiality or

1.D.4.2. The research presents no more than minimal risk and involves no procedures for which written consent is normally required outside of the research context.

1.D.5. The IRB conducts audits to determine that waivers or alterations of informed consent are only made when permitted by regulation.

1.D.5.1. The IRB uses the results for QI purposes and takes action, as needed.

IC 2 The IRB protects human subjects participating in research conducted with exceptions from the informed consent requirements.

Requirement	Element	Data Source	Method

2.A. The IRB has policies and procedures for exceptions from the general requirements for obtaining informed consent before the use of a test article and appropriately reviews such exceptions.
 	
Regulation/Source
21 CFR 50.23
IRB-GB, (III)(B)
FDA-IS, (CL)(XIII)
FDA-IS, (ICG)
	For each individual situation in which a test article is to be administered and informed consent may not feasibly be obtained:
	2.A.1. The IRB requires that the investigator and a physician who is not otherwise participating in the clinical investigation must certify in writing all of the following:
	  2.A.1.1. The subject is confronted by a life-threatening situation necessitating the use of the test article.
	  2.A.1.2. Informed consent cannot be obtained from the subject because of an inability to communicate with, or obtain legally effective consent from, the subject.
	  2.A.1.3. Time is not sufficient to obtain consent from the subject's legal representative.
	  2.A.1.4. There is no alternative method of approved or generally recognized therapy that provides an equal or greater likelihood of saving the life of the subject.
	2.A.2. The IRB requires that if the immediate use of the test article is, in the investigator's opinion, required to
		Policies and procedures for exceptions from the general requirements for obtaining in-formed consent before the use of a test article
		
		IRB minutes
		
		Sample of protocols
		
		IRB Chair interview
		
		QI results
			Review of policies and procedures for evidence of requirements for obtaining informed consent before the use of a test article
			
			IRB minutes document evaluation of each exception to the general requirements for obtaining informed consent
			
			Exceptions to the general requirements to informed consent met all required conditions
			
			Ask the IRB Chair to express conditions for exceptions to the general requirements for obtaining informed consent
			
			QI results show evidence that exceptions to general requirements for obtaining informed consent met required conditions

preserve the life of the subject, and time is not sufficient to obtain the independent determination by a physician not otherwise participating in the study, in advance, the use of the test article shall be reviewed and evaluated within 5 working days in writing by a physician not participating in the investigation.

2.A.3. The IRB requires documentation of emergency situations where exceptions to the general requirements to informed consent have occurred to be submitted to the IRB within 5 working days.

2.A.4. In its review of requests for exceptions, the IRB documents the regulatory basis for the exception and the timely receipt of written certification.

2.A.5. The IRB conducts audits to determine that exceptions from the general requirements for obtaining informed consent before use of a test article are made appropriately.

2.A.5.1. The IRB uses the results for QI purposes and takes action, as needed.

2.B. The IRB has policies and procedures for exceptions from informed consent requirements in planned emergency research and appropriately reviews such exceptions.

2.B.1. The IRB requires planned emergency research proposals include documentation of all of the following:

2.B.1.1. The human subjects are in a life-threatening situation, available treatments are unproven

Policies and Procedures

IRB minutes

Review of policies and procedures for requirements for emergency research exceptions from informed consent requirements

IRB minutes reflect evaluation of

Regulation/Source		Data Source	Evidence
21 CFR 50.24 IRB-GB, (III)(B) FDA-IS, (CL)(XIII) FDA-IS, (ICG)	or unsatisfactory, and the collection of valid scientific evidence is necessary to determine the safety and effectiveness of particular interventions. 2.B.1.2. Obtaining informed consent is not feasible. 2.B.1.3. Participation in the research holds out the prospect of direct benefit to subjects. 2.B.1.4. The clinical investigation could not practically be carried out without the waiver. 2.B.1.5. The proposed investigational plan defines the length of the potential therapeutic window based on scientific evidence and the investigator has committed to attempting to contact a legally authorized representative within that window of time. 2.B.1.6. The IRB has reviewed and approved informed consent procedures and an informed consent document as set forth in VA and other federal regulations to be used in situations where the use of such procedures and documents is feasible. 2.B.1.7. Additional protections of the rights and welfare of the subjects will be provided through, at least, 2.B.1.7.1. Consultation with representatives of the community,	Sample of protocols IRB communications QI results	exceptions from informed consent in planned emergency research Review of protocols for planned emergency research shows evidence of meeting requirements (i.e., public disclosure, plan for subject and family notification, etc.) IRB communications provide evidence of meeting requirements (i.e., public disclosure, plan for subject and family notification, etc.) QI results show evidence of compliance in evaluating and implementing planned emergency research

2.B.1.7.2. Public disclosure to the community prior to the study.

2.B.1.7.3. Public disclosure of the results of the investigation following completion.

2.B.1.7.4. Establishment of an independent data monitoring committee.

2.B.1.7.5. The investigator will summarize efforts made to contact family members and make this information available to the IRB at the time of continuing review.

2.B.1.8. Procedures are in place to inform, at the earliest feasible opportunity, each subject or legally authorized representative or family member, of the subject's inclusion in the clinical investigation.

2.B.1.9. There is a procedure to inform the subject, legally authorized representative, or family member that the subject's participation may be discontinued at any time without penalty or loss of benefits to which the subject is otherwise entitled.

2.B.1.10. There must be a separate IND or IDE for the study for any FDA-regulated product.

2.B.1.11. If the study does not involve an FDA-regulated

194

product, there is concurrence by the Agency Secretary that the waiver is appropriate.

2.B.2. In its review of requests for exceptions in planned emergency research, the IRB documents its evaluation and the regulatory basis for approving the exception.

2.B.3. The IRB conducts audits that include a review of requests for exceptions from informed consent in planned emergence research.

2.B.3.1 The IRB uses the results for QI purposes and takes action, as needed.

Process for Submitting Comments
(due by May 15, 2001)

Please address all comments to VAHRP:

- **E-mail (preferred method)** to **vahrpap@ncqa.org**. You will receive an e-mail confirmation of receipt.

- **Mail** to VAHRPAP, NCQA, 2000 L Street, N.W., Suite 500, Washington, D.C. 20036

- **Fax** to 202-955-3599, Attention – *VAHRPAP.*

Please provide the following information:

- Name

- Position

- Organization

Please organize comments as described below.

- **Word document (preferred method)** formatted as below.

Domain	Issue*	Comment
Privacy and Confidentiality	Requirement 1.B Data source/method	Should the IRB minutes be included as a possible data source/method for evaluating IRB assessment of provisions to protect privacy in individual proposals?
All	Data Source/method	Is a one-year look-back period an appropriate timeframe for adequate evaluation of an HRPP?

* Issue may address a global comment, a specific requirement or element, the data sources or methods

Committee, Expert Adviser, and Staff Biographies

Daniel D. Federman, M.D., *Chair*, is senior dean for alumni relations and clinical teaching and the Carl W. Walter Distinguished Professor of Medicine and Medical Education at Harvard Medical School. He graduated from Harvard College and Harvard Medical School and completed his internship and residency at Massachusetts General Hospital. Dr. Federman conducted research and trained in endocrinology at the National Institutes of Health, the University College Hospital Medical School in London, and Massachusetts General Hospital, where he served as a physician, chief of the Endocrine Unit, and associate chief of medical services. During his 4-year tenure at Stanford University Medical School, he was physician-in-chief, the Arthur F. Bloomfield Professor of Medicine, and chair of the Department of Medicine. In 1977, Dr. Federman returned to Harvard Medical School, where he has held the posts of dean for students and alumni, dean for medical education, and professor of medicine. He has served as chair of the Board of Internal Medicine and president of the American College of Physicians. He is a member of the Institute of Medicine and served on the Committee on Understanding the Biology of Sex and Gender Differences.

Daniel L. Azarnoff, M.D., is president of D. L. Azarnoff Associates and senior vice president of Clinical and Regulatory Affairs of Cellegy Pharmaceuticals. He has more than 20 years of academic experience in research and clinical medicine. For 8 years Dr. Azarnoff served as president of research and development for the Searle Pharmaceutical Company, and for the past 14 years he has served as a consultant in drug development. Before joining Searle he was Distinguished Professor of Medicine and Pharmacology and director of the Clinical

Pharmacology Toxicology Center at the University of Kansas Medical Center, a job he held for 16 years. He has published more than 175 articles in scientific and medical journals. Dr. Azarnoff is a member of the Institute of Medicine and a fellow of the American Association of Pharmaceutical Scientists, the New York Academy of Sciences, and the American College of Physicians, and is chair-elect of the Pharmaceutical Section of the American Association for the Advancement of Science. He maintains a teaching appointment at the schools of medicine of the University of Kansas and Stanford University. Dr. Azarnoff has been on the editorial boards of several journals and on committees of the U.S. Food and Drug Administration, World Health Organization, American Medical Association, National Academy of Sciences, Institute of Medicine, and National Institutes of Health, advising them on drugs and drug development.

Tom L. Beauchamp, Ph.D., is professor of philosophy and senior research scholar at the Kennedy Institute of Ethics. He received graduate degrees from Yale University and the Johns Hopkins University, where he received a Ph.D. in 1970. He then joined the faculty of the Philosophy Department at Georgetown University and in the mid-1970s accepted a joint appointment at the Kennedy Institute of Ethics. In 1976, he joined the staff of the National Commission for the Protection of Human Subjects of Biomedical and Behavioral Research, where he wrote the bulk of *The Belmont Report* (1978). Dr. Beauchamp's research interests are in Hume and the history of modern philosophy and practical ethics, especially biomedical ethics and business ethics. Publications include the following co-authored works: *Hume and the Problem of Causation* (Oxford University Press, 1981), *Principles of Biomedical Ethics* (Oxford University Press, 1979 4th ed., 1994), *A History and Theory of Informed Consent* (Oxford University Press, 1986), and *Philosophical Ethics* (McGraw-Hill, 1982 2nd ed., 1991). Publications also include a number of edited and co-edited anthologies and more than 100 scholarly articles in journals and books. Dr. Beauchamp is the General Editor—with David Fate Norton and M. A. Stewart—of *The Critical Edition of the Works of David Hume*, Clarendon Press, Oxford University Press. He is also the editor of an electronic edition called HUMETEXT (co-editor, David Fate Norton), a complete electronic edition of Hume's philosophical, political, and literary works.

Timothy Stoltzfus Jost, J.D., is the Newton D. Baker-Baker and Hostetler Professor of Law and also a professor of health services management at the College of Medicine and Public Health, Ohio State University. He is the author of a book on comparative health law and a co-author of casebooks in health law and in property law and has published a number of articles concerning health care regulation and comparative health law. Professor Jost has served as a consultant to the Institute of Medicine, the Administrative Conference of the United States, and the American Bar Association's Commission on Legal Problems of the Elderly and was a member of the State of Ohio Medical Board. A recipient of a Western European Regional Research Fulbright Grant, Professor Jost spent the winter and spring of 1989 at the Oxford University Centre for Socio-Legal Studies. He was also a guest professor at the University of Goettingen in Germany on a Fulbright grant in 1996–1997. In 2000, Professor Jost received the Jay Healey Distinguished Health Law Teacher Award from the American Society of Law, Medicine, and Ethics. He earned a B.A. in history at the University of California, Santa Cruz, and a J.D. from the University of Chicago.

Patricia A. King, J.D., is the Carmack Waterhouse Professor of Law, Medicine, Ethics and Public Policy at Georgetown University Law Center. She is also an adjunct professor in the Department of Health Policy and Management, School of Hygiene and Public Health, the Johns Hopkins University, and chair of the board of trustees of Wheaton College. She is the co-author of *Cases and Materials on Law, Science, and Medicine* and an area editor of the *Encyclopedia of Bioethics* (MacMillan Publishing Company). A member of the American Law Institute, she is also a fellow of the Hastings Center and a senior research scholar at the Kennedy Institute of Ethics. She has served on numerous committees of the Institute of Medicine. Her work in the field of bioethics has included service as cochair for policy of the Embryo Research Panel, National Institutes of Health; the U.S. Department of Health, Education, and Welfare Recombinant DNA Advisory Committee; the President's Commission for the Study of Ethical Problems in Medicine and Biomedical and Behavioral Research; the National Commission for the Protection of Human Subjects of Biomedical and Behavioral Research; and the Ethics, Legal and Social Issues Working Group of the Human Genome Project. She is also a member of the boards of the National Partnership for Women and Families and the Hospice Foundation. Before joining Georgetown University, she was the deputy director of the Office of Civil Rights at the U.S. Department of Health, Education, and Welfare and special assistant to the chair of the Equal Employment Opportunity Commission. She also served as a deputy assistant attorney general in the Civil Division of the U.S. Department of Justice. Ms. King received a B.A. from Wheaton College and a J.D. from Harvard Law School.

Roderick J. A. Little, Ph.D., is professor and chair of the Department of Biostatistics of the School of Public Health at the University of Michigan. He has also been a professor in the Department of Biomathematics at the University of California, Los Angeles, School of Medicine and a scientific associate for the World Fertility Survey. Little has been an American Statistical Association/U.S. Bureau of the Census/National Science Foundation research fellow and has held faculty positions at the George Washington University and the University of Chicago. He is a fellow of the American Statistical Association and an elected member of the International Statistical Institute. He received a Ph.D. in statistics from London University's Imperial College. He is currently a member of the National Research Council's Committee on National Statistics. He has expertise in the areas of survey sampling and statistical analysis of incomplete data and has broad experience with applications of statistics to demography, the social sciences, and biomedical research.

James McNulty serves on the board and the Executive Committee of the National Alliance for the Mentally Ill (NAMI), Rhode Island, as well as the Mental Health Consumer Advocates of Rhode Island, a statewide organization for mental health consumers. Having experienced the full impact of mental illness personally, he has been active in involving patient and family advocates in all aspects of treatment of mental illness. Mr. McNulty is a member of the Board of Directors of NAMI National and is president of the Manic Depressive & Depressive Association of Rhode Island. He served on the Protection and Advocacy Program for Persons with Mental Illness advisory committee for Rhode Island, as well as the board of the Rhode Island Protection Advocacy Services Agency. For several years, Mr. McNulty served on the Institutional Review Board of Butler Hospital, a freestanding psychiatric teaching hospital affiliated with the Brown University School of Medicine. He began his service with the Human Subjects Research Council Workgroup of the National Advisory Mental Health Council in 1999. He is a member of the Executive Committee of the Clinical Antipsychotic Trials of Intervention Effectiveness Project, a National Institute of Mental Health-funded multisite research protocol evaluating the efficacy of atypical antipsychotics in schizophrenia and Alzheimer's disease. Mr. McNulty also serves on the Governor's Council on Mental Health in Rhode Island and the National Advisory Mental Health Council.

Anne C. Petersen, Ph.D., has been senior vice president for programs at the W. K. Kellogg Foundation since 1996. Dr. Petersen was deputy director and chief operating officer of the National Science Foundation from 1994 to 1996, the first woman in the agency's 45-year history to serve in that position. She also served as the vice president for research, as well as dean of the Graduate School, at the University of Minnesota. Dr. Petersen has authored many books and articles on adolescence, gender, and research methods and is a fellow of the American Association for the Advancement of Science, the American Psychological Association, and the Institute of Medicine, and is on the Executive Committee of the International Society for the Study of Behavioral Development, among other societies. In addition, she is a member of the National Advisory Mental Health Council at the National Institutes of Health, and Board of Trustees of the National Institute of Statistical Sciences. She holds a bachelor's degree in mathematics, a master's degree in statistics, and a doctorate in measurement, evaluation, and statistical analysis, all from the University of Chicago.

Bonnie W. Ramsey, M.D., is director of the Pediatric General Clinical Research Center and Cystic Fibrosis Research Center at Children's Hospital and Regional Medical Center in Seattle. She is a professor in the Department of Pediatrics and program director, Core Center for Gene Therapy, University of Washington School of Medicine. She also is the director of the Cystic Fibrosis Foundation's newly formed Therapeutics Development Network Coordinating Center. Dr. Ramsey is an active member of several national professional societies including the American Thoracic Society and the American Academy of Pediatrics, serves on the Board of Trustees of the Cystic Fibrosis Foundation, and is chair of the Medical Advisory Committee for the National Cystic Fibrosis Foundation. She also serves as an ad hoc reviewer for the *New England Journal of Medicine, Journal of Pediatrics, Human Gene Therapy, Pediatric Pulmonology,* and *American Journal of Respiratory and Critical Care Medicine.* Dr. Ramsey has served on several government agency advisory panels including the Pulmonary Advisory Board, U.S. Food and Drug Administration, and advisory review groups for the National Heart, Lung, Blood Institute, National Institute of Diabetes and Digestive and Kidney Diseases, and National Center for Research Resources. Dr. Ramsey earned an undergraduate degree from Stanford University and a medical degree from Harvard Medical School.

Lydia Villa-Komaroff, Ph.D., is professor of neurology and vice president for research at Northwestern University, where she is responsible for policy formulation, strategy design, and operational oversight of the research infrastructure. She received an A.B. in biology from Goucher College and a Ph.D. in cell biology from the Massachusetts Institute of Technology. During her research career, she gained international recognition as a molecular biologist and was a key member of the team that first demonstrated that bacterial cells could produce insulin. Dr. Villa-Komaroff was an associate professor of neurology at Harvard Medical School and Children's Hospital and associate director of the Division of Neuroscience at Children's Hospital in Boston. She has published more than 60 articles and reviews and has served on a number of review committees for the National Institutes of Health. She was a member of the Advisory Committee for the Biology Directorate of the National Science Foundation (chair from 1997 to 1998), a member of the congressionally mandated National Science Foundation Committee on Equal Opportunity in Science and Engineering, and an invited participant in the Forum on Science in the National Interest sponsored by the White House Office of Science and Technology Policy. She is a founding member of the Society for the Advancement of Chicanos and Native Americans in Science and has served as a board member and vice president.

Frances M. Visco, J.D., has served as president of the National Breast Cancer Coalition (NBCC), an organization dedicated to eradicating breast cancer through action and advocacy, since its inception in 1991. Ms. Visco is a two-term member of President Bill Clinton's Cancer Panel, chair of the National Action Plan on Breast Cancer, past chair of the National Action Plan on Breast Cancer, and immediate past chair of the Integration Panel of the U.S. Department of Defense Peer-Reviewed Breast Cancer Research Program. After her own successful battle with breast cancer, she began her crusade as a breast cancer activist with the Linda Creed Breast Cancer Foundation. She continues to serve on the board of that foundation and is active in many of its programs. Until April 1995, Ms. Visco was a commercial litigator and partner at the law firm of Cohen, Shapiro, Polisher, Shiekman & Cohen in Philadelphia. Ms. Visco graduated from St. Joseph's University and Villanova Law School. She is serving on the National Cancer Policy Board.

EXPERT ADVISERS

Kay Dickersin, Ph.D., is associate professor, Department of Community Health, Brown University School of Medicine, and codirector of the New England Cochrane Center within the Cochrane Collaboration, which aims to facilitate systematic reviews of randomized controlled trials across all areas of health care. She is also adjunct associate professor in the Department of Epidemiology and Preventive Medicine at the University of Maryland School of Medicine, at the Johns Hopkins University Department of Epidemiology, and at the division of clinical care at Tufts University Department of Medicine. Her primary academic interests are evidence-based medicine, clinical trial design, and meta-analysis. Dr. Dickersin directs the coordinating center for two federally funded, multicenter randomized trials: the Ischemic Optic Decompression Trial and the Surgical Treatments Outcomes Project for Dysfunctional Uterine Bleeding. She is on the Board of Directors for the Society for Clinical Trials and has served on the Institutional Review Board at the Johns Hopkins School of Hygiene and Public Health. From 1994 to 2000 she served on the National Cancer Advisory Board. She received a B.A. and an M.A. in zoology at the University of California, Berkeley, and then earned a Ph.D. in epidemiology at the Johns Hopkins University.

Alberto Grignolo, Ph.D., is senior vice president and general manager for Worldwide Regulatory Affairs at PAREXEL International, a contract research organization, where he is responsible for the company's regulatory services, including worldwide registration strategies and submissions, regulatory compliance, and clinical quality assurance for pharmaceuticals, biologicals, and medical devices. An internationally recognized regulatory professional and public speaker, Dr. Grignolo joined PAREXEL in 1992 as head of worldwide regulatory consulting services. Before going to PAREXEL, he held a series of regulatory and executive management positions at SmithKline Beecham and Fidia Pharmaceutical. A long-standing member of the Regulatory Affairs Professionals Society, he was president and chairman of the board from 1991 to 1992. Dr. Grignolo is currently a member of the Board of Directors of the Drug Information Association (DIA). He is chair of the Regulatory Track of the 2001 DIA Annual Meeting and serves on the Steering Committee of the Americas, the Regulatory Special Interest Advisory Committee, the Marketing Committee, and the Regulatory Training Faculty. Dr. Grignolo holds a Ph.D. in experimental psychology from the University of North Carolina and a B.S. in psychology from Duke University.

Mary Faith Marshall, Ph.D., B.S.N., is professor of medicine and bioethics at Kansas University Medical Center, where she also holds joint appointments in the School of Nursing and Allied Health and the Department of History and Philosophy of Medicine and serves on the Institutional Review Board and the Conflict of Interest Committee. She is principal investigator of the Research Integrity Project at the Midwest Bioethics Center. At the U.S. Department of Health and Human Services she serves as chair of the National Human Research Protections Advisory Committee and as an expert adviser to the Office for Human Research Protections on research involving children and prisoners. At the National Institutes of Health, Dr. Marshall served on the first special research ethics review panel advisory to the director and sits on the Cardiology and Hematology Data Safety and Monitoring Boards of the National Heart, Lung, and Blood Institute. She is a past president of the American Society for Bioethics and Humanities. Dr. Marshall received a B.S.N. and a Ph.D. in religious studies (applied ethics) from the University of Virginia. She has published numerous books, chapters, and articles in the fields of perinatal substance abuse as well as clinical and research ethics.

Carol Saunders, R.N., is president and chief executive officer of the Center for Clinical Research Practice, a corporation that produces and publishes educational and management resources for institutions, sponsors, and clinical research professionals. She is executive director of the New England Institutional Review Board, which provides ethical review services for sponsors and investigators of drug and device studies. Co-editor of *Research Practitioner*, she has published extensively and lectured on a broad range of research-related topics and has been recognized for excellence in medical communications by the American Medical Writers Association. She has co-authored several textbooks on clinical research and human subject protection, including standard operating procedures for investigative sites. She earned a B.S.N. from Boston College and serves as consulting faculty at Duke University.

Dennis Tolsma, M.P.H., is director of the Division of Clinical Quality Improvement and director of research at Kaiser Permanente in Atlanta. He is chair-elect (2001–2002) for the Board of HMO Research Network, chair of the Sci-

ence Steering Committee for a Centers for Disease Control and Prevention research contract with the Alliance for Community Health Programs and America
Association of Health Plans Science Committee, and a member of the Kaiser
Permanente Research Advisory Council. From 1994 to 1998, he was director of
prevention and practice analysis for Kaiser Permanente and chaired the company's Institutional Review Board from 1995 to 1999. Before joining Kaiser, he
was associate director of public health practice at the Centers for Disease Control and Prevention. He received an A.B. in mathematics and English from Cal-
vin College and an M.P.H. from Columbia University.

LIAISONS

Richard J. Bonnie, L.L.B., is John S. Battle Professor of Law at the University
of Virginia School of Law and director of the University's Institute of Law, Psychiatry, and Public Policy. He previously served as associate director of the National Commission on Marijuana and Drug Abuse, a member of the National
Advisory Council on Drug Abuse, chair of Virginia's State Human Rights
Committee responsible for protecting the rights of persons with mental disabili-
ties, adviser for the American Bar Association's Criminal Justice Mental Health
Standards Project, and a member of the John D. and Catherine T. MacArthur
Foundation Research Network on Mental Health and the Law. He was a member
of a delegation of the U.S. State Department that assessed changes in the Soviet
Union relating to political abuse of psychiatry and is a member of the Board of
Directors of the Geneva Initiative on Psychiatry. Mr. Bonnie is a member of the
Institute of Medicine and has also served on and chaired numerous Institute of
Medicine committees. In addition, he serves as an adviser to the American Psy-
chiatric Association's Council on Psychiatry and Law and received the Ameri-
can Psychiatric Association's prestigious Isaac Ray Award in 1998 for contribu-
tions to forensic psychiatry and the psychiatric aspects of jurisprudence. Mr.
Bonnie is a liaison from the IOM Board on Neuroscience and Behavioral
Health.

Nancy Neveloff Dubler, L.L.B., is the director of the Division of Bioethics,
Department of Epidemiology and Social Medicine, Montefiore Medical Center,
and professor of bioethics at the Albert Einstein College of Medicine. She received a B.A. from Barnard College and an LL.B. from Harvard Law School.
Ms. Dubler founded the Bioethics Consultation Service at Montefiore Medical
Center in 1978 as a support for analysis of difficult cases presenting ethical issues in the health care setting. She lectures extensively and is the author of numerous articles and books on termination of care, home care and long-term care,
geriatrics, prison and jail health care, and AIDS. She is codirector of the Certificate Program in Bioethics and the Medical Humanities, conducted jointly by
Montefiore Medical Center, the Albert Einstein College of Medicine, and the

Hartford Institute of Geriatric Nursing at New York University. Her most recent books are *Ethics on Call: Taking Charge of Life and Death Choices in Today's Health Care System*, published by Vintage in 1993, and *Mediating Bioethical Disputes*, published in 1994 by the United Hospital Fund in New York City. She consults often with federal agencies, national working groups, and bioethics centers and served as cochair of the Bioethics Working Group at the National Health Care Reform Task Force. Ms. Dubler is a liaison from the Board on Health Sciences Policy.

Elena Ottolenghi Nightingale, M.D., Ph.D., is a scholar-in-residence at the National Research Council and the Institute of Medicine (IOM) and adjunct professor of pediatrics at both Georgetown University Medical Center and George Washington University Medical Center. Dr. Nightingale serves as liaison or adviser to several IOM activities and is a member emerita of the IOM Board on Health Promotion and Disease Prevention.. For more than 11 years she was special adviser to the president and senior program officer at Carnegie Corporation of New York and lecturer in social medicine at Harvard University. She retired from both positions at the end of 1994. Dr. Nightingale earned an A.B. degree in zoology, summa cum laude, from Barnard College of Columbia University, a Ph.D. in microbial genetics from the Rockefeller University, and an M.D. from New York University School of Medicine. She is a fellow of the American Association for the Advancement of Science, the New York Academy of Sciences, and the Royal Society of Medicine. She has authored numerous book chapters and articles on microbial genetics, health (particularly child and adolescent health and well-being and health promotion and disease prevention), health policy, and human rights. Her current research interest is in improving the safety and security of young adolescents in the United States. Dr. Nightingale continues to be active in the protection of human rights, particularly those of children. She also continues to work on enhancing the participation of health professionals and health professional organizations in the protection of human rights. She has lectured and written widely on these topics, particularly on the role of physicians as perpetrators of human rights violations and as protectors of human rights. Currently she serves on the Advisory Committee of the Children's Rights Division of Human Rights Watch. She has also served on the Board of the Children's Research Institute of the Children's National Medical Center in Washington, D.C., and is on the Institutional Review Board of that institution. Dr. Nightingale is a liaison from the IOM Board on Children, Youth, and Families.

Pilar Ossorio, Ph.D., J.D., is assistant professor of law and medical ethics at the University of Wisconsin at Madison. Before taking this position, she was director of the Genetics Section at the Institute for Ethics of the American Medical Association. Dr. Ossorio received a Ph.D. in microbiology and immunology in 1990 from Stanford University. She went on to complete a postdoctoral fellowship in cell biology at Yale University School of Medicine. Throughout the early 1990s, Dr. Ossorio also worked as a consultant for the federal program on the Ethical, Legal, and Social Implications (ELSI) of the Human Genome Project, and in 1994 she took a full-time position with the U.S. Department of Energy's ELSI program. In 1993, she served on the Ethics Working Group for President Bill Clinton's Health Care Reform Task Force. Dr. Ossorio received a J.D. from the University of California at Berkeley School of Law (Boalt Hall) in 1997. She was elected to the legal honor society Order of the Coif and received several awards for outstanding legal scholarship. Dr. Ossorio is a fellow of the American Association for the Advancement of Science (AAAS), a past member of AAAS's Committee on Scientific Freedom and Responsibility, and a member of the National Cancer Policy Board and has been a member or chair of several working groups on genetics and ethics. She has published scholarly articles in bioethics, law, and molecular biology. Dr. Ossorio is a liaison from the IOM National Cancer Policy Board.

STUDY STAFF

Laura Lyman Rodriguez, Ph.D., is a senior program officer for the Board on Health Sciences Policy at the Institute of Medicine and is the study director for Assessing the System for Protecting Human Research Subjects. She came to the Institute of Medicine from the Office of Public Affairs at the Federation of American Societies for Experimental Biology (FASEB), where she was a policy analyst covering human subjects research and institutional review board issues, bioethics, and federal funding priorities. Before her tenure at FASEB, Dr. Rodriguez was a congressional fellow in the office of Representative Vernon J. Ehlers (R-MI), where she focused on national science policy issues and math and science education from kindergarten through grade 12. Dr. Rodriguez has expertise in cell biology and genetics and is particularly interested in clinical research issues and the policy implications of genomics.

Robert Cook-Deegan, M.D., is a senior program officer for the National Cancer Policy Board, Institute of Medicine (IOM), and Commission on Life Sciences (National Academy of Sciences), and for IOM's Health Sciences Policy Board. He is also a Robert Wood Johnson Health Policy Investigator at the Kennedy Institute of Ethics, Georgetown University, where he is writing a primer on how national policy decisions are made about health research, and a seminar leader for the Stanford-in-Washington program, for which he recently directed a world survey of genomics research.

Jessica Aungst is a research assistant for the Board on Health Sciences Policy of the Institute of Medicine. She received a degree in English with a minor in sociology from the State University of New York, Geneseo. Upon graduating, she moved to Washington, D.C., to work for an international newsletter before joining the Institute of Medicine.

Natasha S. Dickson is a senior project assistant with the National Academy of Sciences' Institute of Medicine in Washington D.C. She is a graduate of St. Augustine Senior Comprehensive Secondary School in Trinidad and Tobago. She gained most of her administrative experience while working as a clerical assistant at the University of the West Indies, St. Augustine, Trinidad. She also worked as an advertising sales representative and freelance reporter for the Trinidad Express Newspapers before moving to the United States in March 2000. She became an administrative receptionist for telecommunications lobbyists Simon Strategies LLC before joining the National Academies in March 2001.

IOM BOARD ON HEALTH SCIENCES POLICY STAFF

Andrew Pope, Ph.D., is director of the Board on Health Sciences Policy at the Institute of Medicine. With expertise in physiology and biochemistry, his primary interests focus on environmental and occupational influences on human health. Dr. Pope's previous research activities focused on the neuroendocrine and reproductive effects of various environmental substances on food-producing animals. During his tenure at the National Academy of Sciences and since 1989 at the Institute of Medicine, Dr. Pope has directed numerous studies. The topics of those studies include injury control, disability prevention, biological markers, neurotoxicology, indoor allergens, and the enhancement of environmental and occupational health content in medical and nursing school curricula. Most recently, Dr. Pope directed studies on priority-setting processes at the National Institutes of Health, fluid resuscitation practices in combat casualties, and organ procurement and transplantation.

CONSULTANT

Kathi E. Hanna, M.S., Ph.D., is a science and health policy consultant specializing in biomedical research policy and bioethics. She has served as research director and senior consultant to the National Bioethics Advisory Commission and as senior adviser to the President's Advisory Committee on Gulf War Veterans' Illnesses. In the 1980s and early 1990s, Dr. Hanna was a senior analyst at the now defunct congressional Office of Technology Assessment, contributing to numerous science policy studies requested by committees of the U.S. House and U.S. Senate on science education, research funding, biotechnology, women's health, human genetics, bioethics, and reproductive technologies. In the past decade she has served as a consultant to the Howard Hughes Medical Institute, the National Institutes of Health, the Institute of Medicine, and several charitable foundations. In the early 1980s, Dr. Hanna staffed committees of the American

Psychological Association that were responsible for oversight of policies related to the protection of human participants in research and animal research. Before coming to Washington, D.C., she was the genetics coordinator at Children's Memorial Hospital in Chicago, where she directed clinical counseling and coordinated an international research program investigating prenatal diagnosis of cystic fibrosis. Dr. Hanna received an A.B. in biology from Lafayette College, an M.S. in human genetics from Sarah Lawrence College, and a Ph.D. from the School of Business and Public Management, George Washington University.

Index

Procedures. *See* Standard operating procedures (SOPs)
Proposed standards, 118–133
    institutional review boards (IRBs), 124–131
    investigators and other research personnel, 131–133
    organizational responsibilities, 118–124
Protection. *See* Human research participant protection programs
Protocol files. *See* Research protocol files
Protocols. *See* Research protocols
Public Responsibility in Medicine and Research (PRIM&R), 1, 6, 8–9, 49–50
    accreditation standards from, 63, 77–80, 115–134
    goals of, 116
    principles underlying protection of humans studied in research, 116–133

Q

Quality improvement (QI) mechanisms, 143
    incorporating continuously into standards, 17, 72

R

Recommendations, 10–20
    for initial standards to begin pilot testing, 84–87
Recruiting research participants, in the draft standards for accreditation of VAMCs, 136, 176–179
Registration process, 52n
Regulatory requirements
    base standards for, 15–17, 71–72
    governmental, 45–46, 71
    relation of standards to existing, 71–72
    rigidity of existing, 55n
Remedial action, draft accreditation outcomes and, 138–140
Repeat accreditation, 53
Research
    inherent risks of, 4
    nonbiomedical, 39–40
    rise of privately funded, 38–39
Research infrastructures, 118, 143
    accommodating a variety of, 13–15, 69–70

Research methods and models, accommodating within accreditation programs, 13–15, 69–70
Research monitoring, 42–43
    improving, 60–61
Research participants/subjects/individuals studied in research, 18n, 118, 142
    directly involving in accreditation programs, 18, 73–75
    in the draft standards for accreditation of VA Medical Centers, 136, 176–179
    naming of, 33–34
    role of, 41–42
    selecting and recruiting, 176–179
    vulnerability of, 144
Research personnel, in proposed standards, 131–133
Research protocol files, 51n, 143
Research protocols, 51n, 143
    conflicts over, 66n
    IRBs evaluating each systematically, 160–167
Risks, 171–175
    considerations of, in the draft standards for accreditation of VA Medical Centers, 136, 171–175
    minimal, 143

S

SAEs. *See* Serious adverse events
Safety reports (IND/IDE), 143
Sanctioning violations, 57–59
Secretary of Health and Human Services, 1, 5
    requesting federal studies for evaluating accreditation, 20, 91–93
    task statement from, 32
Selecting research participants, 176–179
Self-evaluation, accreditation programs and, 51–52
Serious adverse events (SAEs), 143–144
Shutdowns of clinical research, at academic and VA medical centers, 29–31
Social Sciences and Humanities Research Council (Canada), 27
SOP. *See* Standard operating procedure
Special interests, policies required of IRBs with, 129
Sponsors, 41, 118, 144. *See also* Investigator/sponsors